D0938998

The Behavioral Genetics of Psychopathology

A Clinical Guide

RC
455.4
.G4
J36
2005

The Behavioral Genetics of Psychopathology

A Clinical Guide

Kerry L. Jang
University of British Columbia

NYACK COLLEGE MANHATTAN

LAWRENCE ERLBAUM ASSOCIATES, PUBLISHERS
2005   Mahwah, New Jersey   London

Copyright © 2005 by Lawrence Erlbaum Associates, Inc.
All rights reserved. No part of this book may be reproduced in any form, by photostat, microform, retrieval system, or any other means, without prior written permission of the publisher.

Lawrence Erlbaum Associates, Inc., Publishers
10 Industrial Avenue
Mahwah, New Jersey 07430
www.erlbaum.com

Cover design by Kathryn Houghtaling Lacey

Library of Congress Cataloging-in-Publication Data

Jang, Kerry L. (Kerry Leslie), 1962–
    The behavioral genetics of psychopathology : a clinical guide / Kerry L. Jang.
        p. cm.
    Includes bibliographical references and index.
    ISBN 0-8058-4326-4 (alk. paper)
    ISBN 0-8058-5358-8 (pbk.)
        1. Mental illness—Genetic aspects. 2. Behavior genetics. I. Title.

RC455.4.G4J36 2005
616.89'042—dc22   2004042271
                                                              CIP

Books published by Lawrence Erlbaum Associates are printed on acid-free paper, and their bindings are chosen for strength and durability.

Printed in the United States of America
10   9   8   7   6   5   4   3   2   1

Contents

Acknowledgments

Many of the ideas expressed in this book have been shaped by the work of many friends and collaborators over the years, particularly John Livesley, Steven Taylor, and Murray Stein, and I thank them all for sharing. I am sure they will tell me that I have misrepresented or misunderstood them after reading this book, but that will give us another excuse to meet, drink beer, and talk about it.

Special thanks go to Roseann Larstone, my long-suffering assistant who has helped me from the outset of this project to keep track of the many drafts that I regularly misplaced as well as to edit, type, and retype the ones I found. Her language during this time was of a form and style that would make a longshoreman proud. Many thanks to Dr. Bonnie Wiese, who bravely read the first draft and provided invaluable comments on what busy clinicians might care to read about, which helped shape the content of the book.

Finally, a very large thank you to all the career-preparation students from Windermere, Sir David Thompson, John Oliver, Lord Templeton, Sir Charles Tupper, and Lord Byng secondary schools (Vancouver School District) for their diligence in checking and correcting references. I hope the experience has not deterred them from a career in research.

This book was supported, in part, by a New Emerging team Grant (PTS-63186) from the Canadian Institute of Health Research, Institute of Neurosciences, Mental Health and Addiction.

Preface

Nurture depends on genes and genes need nurture.

—Ridley (2003)

This book explores the theories, etiology, measurement, diagnosis, and treatment of psychopathology from the perspective of *behavioral genetics*, a field of enquiry broadly concerned with the inheritance of emotional and behavioral patterns.

Why do clinicians need to know about the new findings being reported every day by behavioral geneticists? The aim of treatment is always to change emotional and behavioral patterns. An understanding of the genetic influences that contribute to behavioral variability and change helps practitioners and patients plan realistic goals and develop effective strategies to reach them. For many people, the term *behavioral genetics* conjures up images of busy automated laboratories searching for susceptibility genes, a job known as *genomics*. With the mapping of the human genome, there is no doubt that genomics will continue to be a large part of what behavioral geneticists do. However, identifying the susceptibility genes is only one effort. The real impact of behavioral genetics lies with studies that estimate the effect of identified or hitherto unidentified genes on behavior, a task that has been labeled *behavioral genomics* (Plomin & Crabbe, 2000). This book addresses the impact of behavioral genomics on how psychopathology is conceptualized and approached in our daily work.

This book is not just about genetics. In February 2001 it was announced that the human genome contains 30,000 genes, rather than the 100,000 originally expected. This startling revision led some to conclude that there are simply not enough genes to account for all the different ways people behave and that behavior must also be shaped by environmental factors. Behavioral geneticists are just as concerned with the influence of the environment and its interplay with genetic factors. This book will try to spend as much time examining the role of experience as biological factors on the development of mental illness.

Inevitably, books on genetics have to log recent findings in the field. However, it is not my intent to simply list results outlining what is genetic and what is not, but rather to try to answer the question, "What does knowing the relative influence of genes and the environment mean at a psychological level of analysis?" What does this mean? This is best answered with an example. It has been argued that diagnostic systems like the *Diagnostic and Statistical Manual of Mental Disorders IV* (American Psychiatric Association, 1994) produce reliable diagnoses of questionable validity, because the system depends on symptom counts to make a diagnosis with little or no mention of the underlying causes of disease (Helmuth, 2003). Behavioral genetics sheds light on these causes, and with a clearer vision of causes we can investigate the validity of current diagnoses, or develop new diagnostic entities based on the degree to which symptoms share a common genetic basis.

This book is divided into nine chapters. The first chapter delineates what behavioral genetics is and what it is not, and the criticisms leveled at the field. This chapter also introduces some ideas on how a biologically based genetic psychopathology is approached with psychotherapy. Chapter 2 is devoted to methods. It describes in basic terms how genetic and environmental effects are estimated and the principal methods used to identify susceptibility genes. Chapter 3 is devoted to diagnosis. This chapter shows how behavioral genetic research challenges the fundamental ideas underlying current nosological and classificatory systems and describes some directions for how they might be revised in the future.

Chapters 4 through 8 review the most common classes of adult psychopathology. Each is a selective survey of the published research in the past decade that provides a sense of what has been studied (as not all forms of psychopathology have come under the behavioral genetic microscope) and how consistent the findings have been. Each highlights one theme that is important in an evolving comprehensive theory of the linkages among genetic influences, environmental factors, and psychopathology.

Chapter 4, on mood disorders, introduces the idea of differential heritability—that psychopathology does not necessarily exist as a monolithic and genetically homogeneous entity, but rather that each symptom is influenced to differing degrees by a multitude of genetic and environmental factors. Chapter 5, on the personality disorders, presents the dimensional model of psychopathology in which illness is conceptualized as the extremes of normal function, and illustrates how behavioral genetics has been used to test the validity of this model.

Of all the psychopathologies discussed in this book, the anxiety disorders have been shown to be influenced by the greatest variety of nonheritable effects. Chapter

6 demonstrates the importance of the environment, specifically, the mechanisms by which the environment (e.g., learning) influence the development of disorder. Chapter 7, on substance use, examines the direct and indirect roles of genetic and environmental effects in alcohol, tobacco, nicotine, and illicit drug use and the relationship between these substances to explain polysubstance use. Chapter 8, on psychotic disorders, traces the ways in which behavioral genetic research has provided support for the neurodevelopmental model of schizophrenia.

The final chapter of this book recapitulates the main findings and also draws attention to new threats to research efforts. I hope that this book helps all readers to make sense of behavioral genetics, and to integrate genetical thinking into daily work, and that it provides a much more informed perspective on mental disorders.

I

Behavioral Genetic Basics

Chapter 1

Introduction

Brain and nervous system disorders may cost the United States as much as $1.2 trillion annually, and affect many millions of Americans each year. Twin data suggest that more than 40% of the societal burden of brain disorders is likely to be genetically mediated. Most of this disease burden arises from complex multigene genetics as well as from environmental influences. The large sizes of these complex genetic burdens should encourage careful molecular and clinical work to link disease vulnerability variants with ... prevention, diagnostics, and therapeutics.

—Uhl and Grow (2004, p. 223)

At first glance, research in behavioral genetics appears to be irrelevant to clinical practice. Rarely do articles comparing the efficacy of different psychotherapeutic approaches make reference to findings in genetics. By the same token, few behavioral genetic research reports discuss the clinical implications of their findings. The independence of science and practice was noted by McClearn, Plomin, Gora-Maslak, and Crabbe (1991), who wrote that, despite the fact that many behavioral geneticists have a background in the social sciences, genetic perspectives on behavior have " ... not yet completely woven into the pattern of psychological theory.... " (p. 222).

An important purpose of this book is to begin the integration of genetics into clinical thinking and research. It is often thought that the only clinical application of genetic research is the development of drug therapies to counteract the offending gene's product. The first major step in this process is to determine if the genes hypothesized to be associated with a disorder are actually present in patients with that disorder. Once a gene is linked to a specific disorder, the biochemistry associated with the gene becomes the focus to determine the intracellular mechanisms by which abnormal behavior is produced. Many researchers in behavioral genetics are trained in medical genetics and other medical specialties. Their approach is to work from the bottom up: They take the fundamental unit of analysis to be the gene and its variants. Frustratingly, successes have been few and far between.

All is not lost, because a great deal of what behavioral geneticists do is to study the effects of these as-yet-to-be identified genes. They take a top down approach that begins with recognized disorders (e.g., the symptoms and signs of mental illness) and uses genetically informative samples, such as twins or adoptees, to determine if individual differences in the disorder are due to genetic variations or to changes in environmental conditions. Genetic effects refer to the influence genes have on the development of individual differences in behavior relative to the influences of learning, experience, and environmental conditions. The size of genetic and environmental effects can be estimated for a single disorder such as major depression or for individual symptoms like sadness or insomnia. We can estimate the relative genetic and environmental impact on virtually any behavior that can be measured reliably. This introductory chapter will explain some important basic concepts, such as the definition of illness, outline some of the criticisms leveled at behavioral genetic research, and finally describe some psychotherapeutic approaches being developed to address behavior whose expression may be fixed by inherited factors.

GENETIC EFFECTS

One of the best-known indices of genetic effect is the *heritability coefficient*, symbolized by the term h^2. This statistic indexes the proportion of the observable differences measured within a sample of people that are directly attributable to the genetic differences between them. Genetic effects are often converted and expressed as percentages. For example, $h^2 = 40\%$ means that 40% of the differences observed between people are directly attributable to genetic differences between them. A popular method to estimate h^2 is to measure the similarities (e.g., using the simple correlation coefficient) of infants who were adopted and raised by biologically unrelated families to their biological family members after they have reached adulthood. Any similarities between the adopted children and their biological relatives can only be due to the genes they share, yielding an estimate of h^2. It follows that if $h^2 = 40\%$, then 60% of the differences between people must be due to environmental factors, including the influence of family environment. Family environmental effects, symbolized as c^2, can be estimated by comparing the similarity of adopted children to their adoptive families. Because they have no genes in common, any similarity can only be due to the fact that they all share the same home environment.

Few disorders are entirely under genetic control. Even if a disorder were 100% heritable, the expression of the relevant genes might still be controlled by environmental factors such as learning experiences or exposure to a specific environmental condition. There are many examples of this phenomenon in the medical literature. An oft-cited example is phenylketonuria (PKU), a form of mental retardation

When R. Adron Harris and his team at the University of Texas, Austin, screened 10,000 genes in the frontal and motor cortexes of alcoholics, they found changes in the expression of 191, they reported in the *Journal of Neurochemistry*.

Alcohol seems to cause a "selective reprogramming" of brain genes in areas involved in judgement and decision making, says Dr. Harris. Among them: genes that code for myelin, whose loss may impair cognition and judgement.

Antidepressants may also alter genes. The conventional wisdom is that drugs such as Prozac work by blocking re-uptake by brain neurons of the neurotransmitter serotonin. But Prozac starts doing that in 24 hours. Why, then, do such drugs typically take weeks to lift depression? "The hunch is that Prozac work by altering gene expression, maybe be causing sprouting of new neurons and remodeling of synapses," Dr. Harris says.

Experience, too, can affect gene expression. How much a mother rat handles and licks off her offspring—an environmental influence if ever there was one—has an astonishing effect: It determines whether genes that code for receptors for stress hormones in the brain are expressed or not. And the level of those receptors affects how a rat reacts to stress. Rats with attentive moms were much less fearful and more curious, finds Michael Meaney of McGill University in Montreal. Rats that got less maternal handling grew up to be timid and withdrawn in novel situations.

Rats are not long-tailed people, so you can't infer that maternal affection affects gene expression and thus temperament in babies, too. But something sure does. There is no shortage of evidence that intelligence, shyness, impulsivity, risk-taking, and illnesses have a genetic component.

But identical twins, who have the same genes, don't have identical traits: One twin might be schizophrenic and the other not, one might be shy and the other outgoing, one might get a "gene-based" cancer and the other not. The difference between identical twins is the experiences they have and, if I may speculate, which of their genes are expressed.

What signal from the environment keeps schizophrenia-related genes silent? What activates IQ-lifting genes? Whatever it is, even a short-lived environmental signal might turn on genes that tell neurons how, and how much to grow. That would leave an enduring mark: Neutral circuits would be complex or simple, and different brain regions would be strongly linked or not. From such neuronal differences arise differences in intelligence and personality, health, and temperament.

Linking specific environmental influences to gene activity would have been a pipe dream only a few years ago. But the new technology of microarray analysis, in which "gene chips" reveal which DNA in a sample of tissue is expressed and which quiescent, is making such discoveries possible.

This past April, in one of their coolest uses so far, gene chips showed that the difference between human brains and chimp brains is not which genes each brain has. Those are nearly identical. The difference is which genes are turned on and which are switched off.

Ironically, the recognition that genes depend on the environment follows hard on the heels of genetics' greatest triumph: sequencing the human genome. But what's now clear is that the more we learn about genetics, the more we'll see that genes are not destiny.

FIG. 1.1. Gene-environment interplay. From "Even Thoughts can Turn Genes 'on' and 'off,'" by S. Begley, June 21, 2002, *San Francisco Chronicle*. Copyright 2003 by the Associated Press. Reprinted with permission from Dow Jones & Company, Inc.

caused by an excess of the amino acid phenylananine. PKU is controlled by the effect of a single gene found on chromosome 12. Inheriting the gene for PKU does not necessarily mean that mental retardation is inevitable. Phenylananine is present in many foods and simply eliminating these foods from the diet of a PKU-gene-carrying infant will prevent the development of genetically mediated mental retardation. This is an example of gene-environment interplay, examples of which can be found for all kinds of human behavior (see Fig. 1.1). Behavioral geneticists have long been awed by the power of the environment and spend as much time and effort identifying these effects as they do in the search for genes and estimating genetic effects.

The Unifactorial Model of Disease

The general public's conception of what constitutes a genetic disease is loosely based on a model of a single gene of major effect—if a person has this gene, they will develop the disease. However, Temple, McLeod, Gallinger, and Wright (2001) described how naïve this popular conception is:

> Human genome sequencing will reveal thousands of genetic variations among individuals that many will assume are associated with disease. But translating such genotypic differences (genetic characteristics) into phenotypic states (visible characteristics) is prone to pitfalls. For example, genetic abnormalities differ in their penetrance (that is, not everyone carrying a genetic abnormality will suffer from adverse consequences); environmental effects have not been taken into consideration; and many diseases have complex etiologies that depend on a number of different genes. There are very few diseases that are caused by a single gene mutation. Automated genomic sequencing is becoming increasingly sophisticated, but distinguishing between normal variations in genes (polymorphisms) and alterations that are detrimental (mutations) remains extremely difficult. This difficulty will have direct consequences for genetic counselors, who must advise individuals about the presence of genetic abnormalities, what they mean, and which treatment or prophylaxis to follow. (pp. 807–808).

The Threshold Liability Model of Disease

How geneticists understand disease is not much different from how behavioral scientists presently conceptualize disorder. This is the classic threshold liability model that assumes that behavior is normally distributed in a population (see Fig. 1.2). The severity of behavior, such as that measured by a self-report or clinical rating scale, is plotted along the horizontal or x-axis. Plotted along the vertical or y-axis is the number of people displaying behavior at a given level of severity. The distribution of scores in this hypothetical population is split into areas representing three distinct groups. The vast majority of people in this population fall within Area A, the normal range of expression. Area B, spectrum conditions, represents the proportion of the population whose behavior does not meet the full criteria to be con-

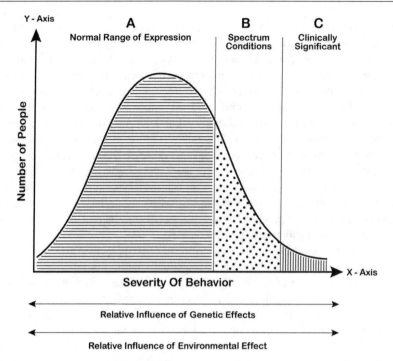

FIG. 1.2.   Threshold liability model of disease.

sidered clinically abnormal (Area C), but is not quite typical enough to be considered normal, that is, fitting the criteria for inclusion in Area A.

The breadth of Areas A, B, and C is defined by the clinician or researcher and need not be symmetrical around the arithmetical average. For example, the point or threshold that differentiates normal from abnormal behavior can be based on statistical criteria (e.g., any score that falls two deviations above or below the mean) or it can be defined as a cut-off on a questionnaire or clinical screen that reliably differentiates patients from healthy controls. For example, clinical research on the Anxiety Sensitivity Index (ASI, Peterson & Reiss, 1992) showed that any score above 25 is clinically significant, irrespective of how the scores are distributed in a population. It is important to remember that, depending on how disorder is defined, it is possible to delineate fewer or more areas (e.g., affected, unaffected vs. unaffected, slightly affected, moderately affected, definitely affected, severely affected) to describe the distribution of disorder in a sample or population.

The threshold liability model is also central in behavioral genetics. However, behavioral geneticists tie severity along the x-axis to the relative influence of genetic and environmental factors that determines the number of people falling into each of the areas. This book presents several ways genetic and environmental influences are thought to increase and decrease the variability of the distribution.

For example, individuals in Area C inherited the specific gene forms for mental illness, had been exposed to the required traumatic events, or were exposed to multiple events over time to cause illness. In contrast, people in Area A did not inherit the genes or may not have been exposed to the requisite traumatic events; people in Area B may have inherited some but not all of the genes for the disorder or have not experienced the critical number or kinds of traumatic events. Alternatively, every person may have inherited the genes that determine susceptibility to disorder, but they remain silent unless triggered into action by exposure(s) to specific environmental stressors or remain silent forever in environments that suppress their actions indefinitely. Similarly, people in Areas A and B may have inherited genes that protect them from the effects of trauma that people in Area C did not inherit. The point is that there are multiple ways genetic and environmental influences work together to produce behavior, that behavior is multifactorial, caused by the action of several genes and experiences.

Other factors that influence the distribution of behavior include the study population (e.g., patient, normal control, general population samples), the sensitivity and specificity of the behavioral measures (e.g., measures that screen for disorders vs. those that assess specific symptoms), and the content of the measure (e.g., designed to assess normal or abnormal behavior). For example, if the study population consisted of unaffected general population study subjects who completed scales that assessed extreme behavior, then there would be no people in Area C, with all falling in Areas A and B. At best, a study based on this population would not be estimating the heritability of a disorder per se, but the heritability of a spectrum condition.

CRITICISMS OF BEHAVIORAL GENETICS

Over the years, a number of objections to behavioral genetic research have been raised, which have no doubt contributed to its apparent lack of impact in clinical circles. Concerns range from questions about the adequacy of research design to the sociopolitical implications of findings. In this section, I offer a brief review of the criticisms and responses, both philosophical and empirical.

Are Heritability Estimates Uninformative?

It is not apparent what scientific purposes are served by the sustained flow of heritability numbers for psychological characteristics. Perhaps molecular geneticists need those numbers to guide their search for underlying genes? Perhaps clinical psychologists need those numbers to guide their selection of therapies that work? Or perhaps educators need those numbers to guide their choice of teaching interventions that will be successful? We have seen no indication of the usefulness of heritability numbers for any of these purposes.... (Kamin & Goldberger, 2002, p. 93)

Is this a valid criticism? It has been argued that the heritability statistic is and has been useful for the very reasons Kamin and Goldberger (2002) suggest. Boomsma, Martin, and Machin (1997) wrote that the raison d'être of twin research was to identify behaviors that would be suitable for genotyping analysis because there is no sense in looking for a susceptibility gene if the disorder is not shown to be heritable in the first place. Moreover, simply demonstrating that a specific behavior is heritable can be paradigm shifting. For example, finding that social attitudes have a substantial heritability challenges the common assumption that they are acquired entirely via social learning (see Olson, Vernon, Harris, & Jang, 2001). Most importantly, it must be remembered that h^2 is just the starting point. Estimating genetic effects on a single variable is the first step to estimating the heritability of a second variable that leads to estimating whether these genetic effects are common to both variables, and this information can be used to explain why behaviors coaggregate the way they do.

Are Behavioral Genetic Methods Inherently Flawed?

One of the classic ways heritability is estimated is by comparing similarities of monozygotic (identical) twins who were separated at birth and raised in different families. This comparison provides a direct estimate of genetic effect because these twins share 100% of their genes but grew up in different environments and any similarities can only be due to their genetic similarity, thus yielding a direct estimate of h^2. Kamin and Goldberger (2002) questioned the validity of heritability estimates based on this method because of concerns over:

1. **The representativeness of samples.** Are the results of studies of twins generalizable to the general population? Do twins live in unique circumstances and receive special treatment from others because they are twins?
2. **The accuracy of the data.** This includes issues about the reliability and validity of self-report versus observer reports and the extent of contact between separated twins. They noted that most behavioral genetic studies rely on self-report questionnaires and often the responses to only a few items from a scale.
3. **Measurement of selective placement effects.** For example, the similarity of twins would be spuriously inflated if twins were placed in homes of families that were genetically similar (e.g., placement based on ethnicity).

It would be fair to characterize these concerns as very much yesterday's news. Behavioral geneticists have addressed them and a large body of relevant research was summarized in Boomsma et al., (1997), an article that, incidentally, predates Kamin and Goldberger's critique by 5 years but was not cited by them. However, the fact that the criticisms continue to be repeated indicates that behavioral geneticists have not done a very good job of publicizing their efforts.

It is also important to point out that some of the criticisms are not unique to behavioral genetic research. For example, the complaint that many studies rely on self-report measures is one that can be leveled at all kinds of behavioral research. In fact, the behavioral genetic research on psychiatric disorders typically uses data collected by clinical interview and other-report (e.g., from parents, roommates, spouses, or teachers) in addition to long and short forms of many popular self-report scales. The choice of instrument used in any study tends to reflect the training of the researcher or its recognition as the best way to measure a particular psychopathology. What the reader should look for is a convergence in results across studies regardless of a scale's response format.

Are Behavioral Geneticists Eugenicists?

Perhaps some of the resistance to behavioral genetics stems from the field's apparent association with the eugenics movement and the spectre of selective breeding of humans for desirable traits. The association began with the publication of Arthur Jensen's 1969 article in the *Harvard Educational Review*, in which he presented early behavioral genetic research that showed that cognitive ability (IQ) had a large heritable component. These findings led some to reason that, if differences in mental abilities are inherited and if success requires those abilities and if earnings and prestige depend on success, then social standing will be based to some extent on inherited differences among people (Bernstein, 1971, p. 43).

People quickly rallied against the IQ test and anything associated with it. A typical response was: "The intelligence test has been used more or less consciously as an instrument of oppression against the under-privileged—the poor, the foreign born and racial minorities" and "a critical review of the literature produces no evidence which would convince a prudent man to reject the hypothesis that intelligence test scores have zero heritability" (Kamin, 1974, p. 1), setting the stage for the sociopolitical "nature versus nurture" battle that has been associated with behavioral genetics ever since.

However, as early as the late 1970s it was clear to many that behavioral genetics was not associated with either side in this debate. For example, Charles Crawford (1979) wrote a tightly argued paper entitled "George Washington, Abraham Lincoln and Arthur Jensen: Are they compatible?" Crawford demonstrated that taking either a pronature or pronurture position was irrational and that the emotion the debate generates stems from the conflict between basic American values and the truth of scientific research.

Crawford (1979) began by describing two core values of American society. The first is that truth despite the consequences is an essential element in the ascent of humanity, exemplified by George Washington's statement: "Father, I cannot tell a lie, I did it with my little hatchet." The second is exemplified by Abraham Lincoln's (reputed) statement that, "If my father's son can become President, so can your father's son." This is no less than the expression of the American dream, which says that, with hard work and determination, anything is possible. The conflict arises because one cannot believe in equal access to the American dream and the inheritance of individual differences in intelligence while maintaining the importance of truth! More importantly, Crawford showed that (see Fig. 1.3) "correctly believing in an

Belief	Possible state of nature	
	Individual differences in intelligence are largely genetic in origin	Individual differences in intelligence are largely environmental in origin
Individual differences in intelligence are largely environmental in origin	Type II error[a] Possible consequences: Individuals encouraged to attempt tasks that some of them cannot master, leading to frustration, guilt, aggression caused by failure Belief in untrue American Dream	Correct decision Possible consequences: Cultural imperialism Equal access to American Dream Orwell's *1984*; Huxley's *Brave New World*
Individual differences in intelligence are largely genetic in origin	Correct decision Possible consequences: Social Darwinism Socialized medicine, guaranteed Annual income, etc. Inventing new American Dream	Type I error[b] Possible consequences: Inappropriate special schools for minority groups Inappropriate marriage, adoption, and miscegenation laws Waste of intellectual talents of many citizens

[a] This would consist in incorrectly believing in environmental determination of individual differences in intelligence.

[b] This would consist in incorrectly believing in genetic determination of individual differences in intelligence.

FIG. 1.3.   Possible consequences of outcomes of the nature-nurture debate. From "George Washington, Abraham Lincoln, and Arthur Jensen: Are They Compatible," by C. B. Crawford, 1979, *American Psychologist, 34*, pp. 664–672. Copyright © 1979 by American Psychological Association. Used with permission.

environmental outcome does not necessarily lead to Utopia in our grandchildren's day and correctly believing in a hereditarian outcome does not necessarily lead to social Darwinism" (p. 664).

Dean Hamer and Peter Copeland came to the same conclusion in their 1998 book *Living With Our Genes*. In this book, they examined what was known about inheritance of everyday human behaviors, including sex, alcohol and drug use, violence, eating habits, and personality. They too found that a polemical debate was pointless and concluded that the "DNA map offers the possibilities and predictions but no certainty" (p. 308), but cheekily added "free will is alive and well, and probably genetic" (p. 314). Behavioral geneticists have never taken the extreme position that heritability equals inevitability and they actively research the role of environmental factors. Among behavioral geneticists, there is simply no debate and the research is not driven by ideology!

GENETICAL PSYCHOTHERAPY

Behavioral genetics examines the effect of genes at the level of populations and samples, but what does a heritable disorder mean at the level of an individual? At this level, genetic predispositions likely impose limits on the degree to which change is possible and the goals of treatment are to help individuals adapt to their psychopathology and express it in useful (or at least neutral) ways. Weinberg (1989) put it best: "Genes do not fix behavior. Rather, they establish a range of possible reactions to the range of possible experiences that environments can provide" (p. 101).

Psychotherapeutic approaches tend to focus on psychosocial adversity and emphasize manipulating the environmental conditions, behaviors, or cognitions to effect change. Many models of psychotherapy are based on the underlying notion that psychopathology is the result of a deficit or conflict. In the deficit model of psychopathology, disorder is characterized by deficits that occurred because the early environment failed to provide the necessary ingredients for the child to develop psychologically. Change is believed to arise from the provision of a supportive, empathic, and validating therapeutic environment. In contrast, traditional psychoanalytic approaches exemplify the conflict model of psychopathology, in which disorder results from defenses against conflicts. The model is attractive because it provides a comprehensive explanation of the development of disorder and simultaneously offers a coherent therapeutic approach. If disorder arises from conflict, it follows that resolution of the conflict using traditional strategies such as confrontation, clarification, interpretation, and working through conflicts, especially in the transference situation, should effect change.

Both models are strongly environmentalist and assert that psychosocial adversity is the major contributing factor. Genetic effects are acknowledged, but have little practical impact on a therapist's concepts of psychopathology that would in turn influence understanding mechanisms of therapeutic change and the goals of therapy. How can knowledge about genetic effects be meaningfully integrated into traditional psychotherapeutic practice? Livesley (2001) suggested that conflict and deficit models need to be supplemented with a vulnerability model of psychopathology that explicitly recognizes genetic predispositions. It postulates that genetic predispositions toward certain illnesses will always exist and that these also impose limits on the degree to which change is possible. The underlying principle of the model is that the combination of genetic predisposition, environmental adversity, and evolving dispositional factors support each other and lead to a system that is "stably unstable."

As such, the goals of therapy are to modify the level of behavioral expression by either dampening or amplifying the effects of genetic predispositions and to influence the selection of behaviors through which psychopathology is expressed. For example, sensation seeking is a highly heritable personality trait. However, not everyone with a high score on sensation seeking will express this trait in the same way, nor will different expressions be equally maladaptive. Maladaptive expressions might include generating excitement by taking an overdose and calling the paramedics or creating public turmoil by threatening to harm oneself or others. More adaptive expressions might include engaging in high-risk sports or speculating on the financial markets as a hobby. Three basic strategies for managing inherited psychopathology are suggested by the model: (a) increasing tolerance and acceptance, (b) attenuating expression, and (c) progressively substituting more adaptive behaviors (Livesley, 1999, 2001).

Increasing Tolerance and Acceptance

The basic premise of this strategy is that behavior is relatively fixed and individuals need to learn to accept their major behavioral characteristics and use them adaptively. Many patients express extreme dissatisfaction and distress about their personal qualities. They attack themselves for having certain characteristics, make war on themselves, in effect. Helping patients to understand that their behavior is inherited and to recognize that most behavior can be adaptive in some way may reduce this internal conflict. Acceptance helps to reduce distress, prevent escalation, and free the individual to use these fixed behaviors constructively.

Livesley (2001) argued that implementing this strategy requires three tasks of the therapist. The first is helping patients understand the core behaviors that define their psychopathology and the factors that lead to the development of these characteristics. The second is helping patients to identify adaptive features of their behavior. Many common behavioral extremes probably emerged during the course of evolution because they conferred some kind of adaptive advantage, but in the present context may no longer do so (e.g., Tooby & Cosmides, 1990). Patients may begin to accept their behavior rather than fight it if they recognize its adaptive potential. The therapist can encourage patients to consider the costs and benefits of their behavior. In the process, maladaptive expressions may be modified and the patient may begin to recognize ways in which the behavior can be useful. Third, reducing the focus on change and identifying relevant situations and activities allows patients to use their basic traits as assets. Gatz (1990) referred to this as creating or localizing a patient's "comfort zone."

Attenuate Expression

The focus in this strategy is teaching patients skills to regulate and control fixed behavior. It assumes that the most malleable component of behavior is the cognitive component and that a cognitive-behavioral approach would be the most useful way to modify maladaptive cognitive strategies that amplify behavioral expression. Beliefs such as "I can't cope with feelings," "My feelings are always out of control," or "There's nothing I can do to stop my feelings" can be challenged and reframed. With other behaviors it may be possible to teach skills that are complementary or incompatible with the behavioral traits, such as stress management and relaxation training. These methods are best introduced gradually (e.g., starting with simple relaxation methods) because many patients find more complex relaxation training aversive.

Progressively Substituting More Adaptive Expression

The assumption in this strategy is that the maladaptive behaviors are relatively fixed but the mode of expression may be changed. For example, patients who exhibit extreme submissive and dependent behaviors can be taught assertiveness skills. This behavioral approach, coupled with efforts to change their beliefs about submission, teaches patients to develop appropriate ways to solicit help and support.

The vulnerability model complements traditional approaches to psychotherapy. All therapists can benefit from an appreciation of the limited extent to which maladaptive behavior may be eradicated in a person; the goal becomes adaptation and control. This can be achieved using standard psychotherapeutic techniques such as cognitive restructuring, counseling or insight, and catharsis. The vulnerability model differs from others only in its explicit recognition of the role of genetics in setting limits on the degree to which behavior can be changed.

SUMMARY

Behavioral genetics research has explored the impact of genes and the environment on disorder. Its results have a direct bearing on our understanding of what psychopathology is and in turn influence our understanding of therapeutic change and the goals of therapy. The next chapter reviews the methods used by behavioral geneticists to estimate genetic and environmental effects and those used to identify genetic loci underlying psychopathology.

Chapter 2

The ABCs of Behavioral Genetics

Underlying all behavioral genetic study designs is the principle that relatives share genes and the additional fact that some relatives, such as siblings, share more genes with each other than with their cousins helps us determine whether heredity is implicated in a disorder. This chapter introduces the ways in which behavioral geneticists find and estimate the effects of genes and the environment. It gives readers sufficiently detailed information on methods and statistics used in the field to enable them to digest and critically appraise the behavioral genetic research reported in the major journals, and to evaluate its implications for their patients.

FINDING GENES

Estimating Genetic Risk

The first step in the search for genes is to identify families in which the risk of developing the disorder is high compared to families randomly sampled from the general population. Risk for a disorder is greater than zero when the frequency of diagnosis is greater among genetically related individuals than in a sample of matched controls. These disorders are also said to be "familial" because they have been shown to "run in families."

Two kinds of genetic risk are commonly estimated using traditional case-control family studies: relative risk (RR) and population relative risk (PRR). These estimates are used to identify high-risk families to be included in gene-hunting studies and in genetic counseling that helps patients and their families make informed choices about marriage and childbearing. RR estimates the extent to which a relative of an affected individual is more likely to develop the condition than a relative of a nonaffected individual. PRR estimates the chances that the relatives of an affected individual are more likely to be affected than the relatives of a nonaffected individual. An example of estimating RR and PRR is presented in Figure 2.1. It is important to remember that these risk estimates also reflect environmental influences on the disorder. Nongenetic factors such as home environment, culture, and frequency of contact also contribute to the similarities between people from the same family. The traditional case-control family design cannot separate the influence of shared genes from shared environmental factors.

Once the high- and low-risk families have been identified and blood samples have been taken from each member, DNA is extracted and the relationship between the DNA and observed behavior is estimated. A generic term for any kind of study that uses DNA analysis is *molecular genetic study*. Molecular genetic studies are designed to tie variations on a specific gene identified in each person's DNA to variations in that person's observable behavior (e.g., presence or absence of the diagnosis or variation on psychological test scores).

	Relatives of schizophrenic individuals	Relatives of controls	Total
N Relatives with Schizophrenia	9	2	11
N Relatives without Schizophrenia	91	98	189
Total	100	100	200

Computing Risk

Relative Risk (RR) = (9/100) + (2/100) = 4.5

Thus a relative of a schizophrenic patient is 4.5 times more likely to become affected with the disease than the relative of a nonschizophrenic patient.

Population Relative Risk (PRR) = (9/100) + (0.15) = 6.0

For this example, we have assumed that the prevalence of the disorder in the general population is 1.5%.

Thus, the relatives of a schizophrenic patient are 6 times more likely to develop the disease than the relatives of a nonschizophrenic patient.

FIG. 2.1.   Computing relative risk and population relative risk. Adapted from "Analysis of Genetic Data: Methods and Interpretation," by R. M. Cantor and J. I. Rotter (Eds.), 1992, The Genetic Basis of Common Diseases (pp. 49–70). Oxford: Oxford University Press. Adapted with permission.

The Linkage Study

One of the primary molecular genetic methods is linkage analysis. Linkage methods use the known locations of genes as road signs or markers for the disease gene to obtain an approximate idea of where it is located on a chromosome. For example, if the disease gene is thought to be on a particular chromosome, a known gene on that chromosome is selected as a marker. The marker may or may not be related to the disease gene. Common markers are blood group genes. According to Mendel's law of genetics, the transmission of genes from parent to offspring should be random. Thus, if the disease gene and marker gene were far apart or on different chromosomes, the probability that they would be passed down together from parent to offspring is zero. Conversely, if the disease gene is physically close to the marker gene, the likelihood that the disease and marker genes would be transmitted together is high and they are said to be *linked*.

The term *linkage* refers to the fact that when genes are in close physical proximity they literally exchange genetic material during meiosis. The exchange of genes from different chromosomes leads to the production of offspring that have a different combination of genes from either parent. The probability of two genes, such as the disease and marker genes, undergoing recombination is called the *recombination fraction*, or θ. This fraction varies from zero to .50. The recombination fraction can be thought of as the distance between the disease and marker genes: A θ of zero indicates close linkage, .30 represents weak linkage, and .50 represents no linkage. In simple terms, θ indexes the degree to which the disease and marker genes are shared among family members of an affected person.

Another statistic, called the *LOD score* (log probability ratio score), is used to estimate the actual likelihood that a disease and marker gene will be transmitted together in a high-risk family. The LOD score is computed as:

$$\text{LOD} = \log 10 \text{ x} \quad \frac{\text{Likelihood of observed pedigree with } \theta < .50}{\text{Likelihood of observed pedigree with } \theta = .50}$$

The LOD score indexes the probability of any observed linkage between disease gene and marker gene in the family tree of an affected person (thus θ will have an actual estimated value of less than .50 in the high-risk family) divided by the probability that any linkage in the family tree is due to chance (hence, θ = .50). If the observed probability of linkage equals the probability that the linkage is due to chance, a LOD score of 1.0 would result, indicating that the level of observed linkage is no different from that expected by chance. If the observed probability of linkage is greater than the probability that the linkage is due to chance, the LOD score would be > 1.0. LOD scores of 3.0 are traditionally considered the statistically significant threshold to indicate that the disease and marker genes are truly linked.

There are three considerations that set limits on the ability of linkage analysis to localize the genes for behavior. First, the method works best when relatively few genes with large effect are implicated in the disorder under study. However, it is currently thought that behavior is actually multifactorial, or caused by the action of several genes of small effect. Second, linkage requires that the affected status of each member of a family can be assigned unequivocally. Any misdiagnosis, whether caused by poor assessment methods, uncertainty or lack of specificity in diagnostic criteria, or the presence of a comorbid disorder—even in a single family member—can have enormous impact on the LOD score. Finally, linkage studies require complete data. The results are jeopardized if some members of the family are unwilling to participate or if data is missing (e.g., affected status of a long-dead relative is unknown).

The Association Study

Association studies have become very popular in the search for susceptibility genes because they do not rely on family pedigrees. Association studies test whether the hypothesized disease gene (or form of a gene called a *polymorphism*) is found in more affected than nonaffected individuals. The method got its name because measures of association such as the correlation coefficient are the primary statistics used to relate genes to behavior. A nice feature of association methods is that they are readily adapted to handle the many different ways behavior is measured in clinical and research settings. For example, by using different correlation coefficients, qualitative (e.g., presence or absence of illness) or quantitative data can be analyzed with equal ease. The strength of the method lies in its use of continuously distributed quantitative data (such as scores on a depression rating scale), where the disorder is measured with enough sensitivity to discriminate between a number of levels of severity. Association studies using quantitative data are referred to as *quantitative trait loci*, or QTL, analyses (see Plomin, DeFries, Craig, & McGuffin, 2003; Plomin & Caspi, 1998 for a detailed review of QTL methods).

Unlike linkage studies, association studies do not pick road signs to localize the position of a disease gene on a chromosome. Rather, they require that the gene selected for analysis actually be involved in the disorder of interest. For example, clinical studies suggest that the neurotransmitter dopamine is implicated in bipolar disorder and any one of several genes active in dopamine production, transport, and reception can be selected for analysis. These are called *candidate genes*.

Candidate genes are also selected on theoretical grounds. For example, Robert Cloninger (1986, 1994) developed the "Biosocial Model of Personality" to provide guidance in the selection of candidate genes. He hypothesized that there are four traits of temperament: harm avoidance, novelty seeking, reward dependence, and persistence. Specific inherited monoamine neurotransmitter systems underlie each trait: serotonin for harm avoidance, dopamine for novelty seeking, and norephinephrine for reward dependence. The model has yet to hypothesize a system for persistence. One of the very first reports of finding a personality gene was a direct result of this model. Cloninger, Adolfsson, and Svrakic (1996) reported a significant association between different forms of the dopamine DRD4 gene and scores on measures of novelty seeking.

The success of association studies greatly depends on identifying a plausible candidate gene. In the absence of a suitable candidate, a systematic and mechanistic approach called the *genome scan* can be used to identify possible candidates. A genome scan associates a number of genes from every chromosome (e.g., every gene that sits 10 centimorgans apart[1]) with disease status. The limitation of genome scans is that they require very large sample sizes of affected people and independent replications to reduce the number of false-positive results one would get by testing so many genes.

As with the linkage study, this method works best when the disease status of people in the study is not confounded by comorbid psychiatric conditions. However, unlike the linkage study, association studies do not require candidate genes with large effects. Association studies have been very successful in identifying polymorphisms that have very small effects, accounting for between 3% and 5% of the variation with acceptable levels of statistical certainty.

In summary, linkage and association studies are designed to localize and identify susceptibility genes for mental illness. The identification of genes and their action will have major implications for drug development. However, the results of these studies are compromised when specific methodological requirements are not met, such as quality of diagnosis (e.g., no misdiagnosis or presence of diagnosed or undiagnosed comorbid conditions) or availability of all family members. At this time, these studies can only estimate the effect of one gene at a time and the results to date suggest that they individually have only a very small effect on behavior.

THE EFFECTS OF GENES AND THE ENVIRONMENT

The heritability coefficient introduced in chapter 1, h^2, is just one of a family of genetic and environmental effects estimated in behavioral genetics research. Figure 2.2 presents a summary of the major effects outlined by Douglas Falconer (1960) in the classic work *Introduction to Quantitative Genetics*. This equation simply states that individual differences observed on a measured behavior (often referred to as the *phenotype*) is attributable to the sum of the genetic (G) and environmental (E) differences between people, in addition to differences caused by the interplay of genetic and environmental factors (GE), and error of measurement. Measurement error is assumed to be random and encompasses the vagaries of the clinical "hunch" to the degree a scale is unreliable.

The term G refers to the variability in observed behavior that is attributable to all sources of genetic influence indexed by h^2_B, commonly referred to as *broad heritability coefficient*. The h is for heritability and the subscript $_B$ is for broad. The

---

[1]A centimorgan, or cM, is a measure of distance between two genetic loci on a chromosome. Two genetic loci are 1 cM apart if their probability of recombination is 1%.

Behavior $X = G + E + GE +$ error

Differences in measured behavior X between people are caused by:

Behavior X = Genetic Differences Between People

+ Environmental Differences Between People

+ The Interplay of Genes and the Environment

+ Errors in Measuring Behavior X

FIG. 2.2. Quantitative genetic theory.

h is squared as a consequence of its computation (described later), but also as a reminder that the quantity is a *variance*. In most statistical textbooks this is symbolized as a squared term such as σ^2 when describing a population, or s^2 when referring to a sample drawn from a population.[2] Heritability estimates index the percentage of the total variation observed on behavior based on all forms of genetic differences between people.

h^2_B subsumes three types of genetic effect: additive genetic effects (h^2_A), genetic dominance effects (h^2_d, and genetic epistasis (h^2_i). Additive genetic effects are those that are passed down directly from parent to offspring. Genetic dominance and epistasis are called "nonadditive" because their effects are not direct but are rather due to the interaction of genes. Genetic dominance is variation attributable to the interaction of genes that occupy the same loci on different chromosomes. An example of genetic dominance effects is the color of a child's hair that is somewhere between the two parents'. Genetic epistasis is caused by the interaction of genes from different loci. Estimates of h^2_i have been difficult to detect because they have been considered small (e.g., Plomin, DeFries, & McClearn, 2000).

How to Estimate Heritability

The first step in measuring any genetic or environmental effect is to measure the similarity of relatives. Similarity is measured by the correlation coefficient, r. Several types of correlation coefficients are used in behavioral genetic research, the type being dictated by several factors including the level of measurement of the instruments used (e.g., dichotomous "yes" = 1 and "no" = 0; continuous or quantitative measures). The type of correlation coefficient, be it the intraclass correlation, Pearson's r, Kendall's g, or Spearman's r, among others, is almost always specified and justified in research reports.[3]

The Adoption Study.   A common way to estimate h^2_B is to compare children who are adopted at birth and raised by genetically unrelated individuals. The

---

[2]Variances are computed as the average of the sum of the squared differences between a person's score from the population or sample average.

[3]In this book, I symbolize all correlations (unless otherwise specified) as r for simplicity.

comparison of the adopted children with their biological parents provides the basis for an estimate of h^2_B because any measured similarity can only be based on genetic similarity (parents and offspring share 50% of the same genetic material on average). Environmental factors cannot contribute to the similarity of the adopted children and their biological parents because members of an unrelated family raised the children.

In this design, estimates of h^2_B are compromised by three factors. The first is that in many modern adoptions the birth mother often maintains some contact with her child and the adoptive family. The degree of contact confounds any estimate of genetic similarity with environmental factors. A second factor is selective placement of adoptees in families with similar backgrounds. For example, it is the policy of many adoption agencies to try to place children of a particular ethnicity into families of the same ethnicity. In this situation, the potential of the birth parents sharing genes with the adoptive family is increased. The risk is higher than one may think. Often, people of the same ethnicity can trace their ancestries back to common cities, towns, or counties in their ancestral homelands and find that their families have intermarried for generations. Third, the ability of researchers to locate sufficient numbers of birth parents to compute the birth parent-offspring comparisons is a concern. If birth parents are not available, heritability estimates can still be computed by comparing siblings who have been placed in different adoptive homes. These families are now quite rare because many jurisdictions have policies to ensure that all children from the same family are adopted into a single home.

The Twin Study.   A straightforward way to estimate h^2_B is to compare the similarity of identical or monozygotic (MZ) twin pairs who were separated at birth and raised apart. Any similarities between raised-apart MZ twins can only be due to their shared genes. Moreover, unlike adoptee siblings, twins are matched for age, which effectively removes any generational differences as a possible source of error.[4] In this design, the computation of h^2_B is accomplished by correlating scores on the behavioral measure between the siblings in each pair. If the correlation is .40, this would mean that 40% of the individual differences on this measure are due to genetic differences between the twin pairs.

Finding sufficient numbers of MZ twins raised apart is difficult, so studies of twins reared together have become the most popular behavioral genetic study design, mainly because of ease of recruitment: Twins who were raised together are relatively plentiful (most national censuses and birth record surveys suggest that twins make up about 2% of the total population) and they tend to keep in touch with one another. Estimating h^2_B on behavior is accomplished by comparing the similarity of MZ twins on the behavior of interest to the similarity of fraternal or dizygotic (DZ)

---

[4]It has been argued that being the first child out of the womb may have some kind of beneficial impact, rendering age differences important. However, there has been little empirical research published to date showing that the effect is significant or important to the development of psychological problems.

twin pairs. Genetic effects are suggested if the similarity of MZ pairs is found to be greater than that of DZ pairs. Figure 2.3 demonstrates how h^2_B is estimated using data from twins who were reared together.

Estimating the Influence of the Environment

Shared Family Environment.   Returning to Fig. 2.2, the term *E* represents all sources of environmental influence on observed individual differences in behavior. Environmental influence is subdivided into two broad classes. The first is the *shared* or *common* environment, symbolized by the statistic c^2, where the *c* refers to the environment (events, conditions, and experiences) that is common to all members in a household. These effects include virtually anything that causes members from the same family to become more similar to one another. Like the heritability estimate, c^2 is a variance that indexes the proportion of the variability in behavior due to differences in family environment between households in a population. A frequently used example of c^2 is total family income measured in dollars. The degree to which a family is above or below the poverty line affects each person within the family in the same way, but differentiates between families in a sample.

The presence of c^2 is readily ascertained in most behavioral genetic designs. For example, in the adoption or twins-reared-apart design the correlation of adoptees with their adoptive parents yields an estimate of the influence of c^2. Any similarity between the adopted child and adoptive parents can only be due to sharing the same family environment. Computation is a little more compli-

---

Twin Correlations   The source of the similarity between twins

Step 1. Twin Similarities

$r_{MZ} =$ .43 100% genes + 100% common family environment

$r_{DZ} =$ .31 50% genes + 100% common family environment

Step 2. Comparing Twin Similarities

$r_{MZ} - r_{DZ} =$ .12 50% genes + 0% common family environment

Step 3. Estimating All of the Genetic Influence

$2 (r_{MZ} - r_{DZ}) = .24$ 2 x 50% = 100% genes estimated

Step 4. Converting to a Proportion

$h^2_B = .24$ x 100% = 24%

24% of the individual differences in behavior *X* is due to all of the genetic differences between people.

FIG. 2.3.   Estimating heritability.

cated in the twins-reared-together design. Here, the MZ correlation is attributable to the fact that both members of each pair share 100% of their genetic endowment and grew up in the same home. In order to estimate c^2, h^2_B must be estimated first and then subtracted from the MZ correlation, leaving an estimate of the proportion of the variance due to common family environment. Figure 2.4 illustrates how c^2 is estimated.

Nonshared Environment.   Although the similarity of MZ twins with respect to major physical characteristics like height or weight is quite high, the correlations are not perfect. MZ twins raised together may share all of their genes and grow up in the same home, but the correlations between them have been shown to fall well below 1.0. What factor accounts for measured differences between identical twins raised together? Assuming that the home environment is the same for both, each must have had unique experiences. This kind of environmental effect is called the *nonshared environment,* symbolized as e^2.

Nonshared environmental influences are defined as any experience, milieu, or circumstance that causes children from the same family to be dissimilar. It would be incorrect to characterize nonshared environmental influences as solely random (e.g., one twin is involved in a motor vehicle accident and the other is not); they can also be experiences that systematically differentiate people (e.g., parents systematically favor one over the other). Figure 2.5 illustrates the computation of e^2 in a reared-together twin design. From this example, the nonshared environmental influence is what remains after genetic similarity and common environmental factors are removed. It is important to remember that estimates of e^2 may be inflated by errors of measurement. If, for example, a clinical interview on one twin was done normally, whereas the interview for the other was rushed, measurable differences might translate into inflated estimates of e^2.

Estimation of the magnitude of shared environmental effects c^2 using Falconer's method.

If $h^2_B = 24\%$ *(from Fig. 2.3) and* $r_{MZ} = .43$ then

$$c^2 = r_{MZ} - h^2_B$$
$$= .43 - .24$$
$$= .19$$
$$= 100 \times .19$$
$$= 19\%$$

Thus, 24% of the individual differences in a measured behavior is due to all of the genetic differences between people; 19% is due to environmental differences between families.

FIG. 2.4.   Estimation of the magnitude of shared environmental effects c^2 using Falconer's method.

Estimation of the magnitude of nonshared environmental effects e^2 using Falconer's method.

If $h^2_B = 24\%$ *(from Fig. 2.3) and* $r_{MZ} = .43$ then
$e^2 = 100 - h^2_B - c^2$
$\quad = 100\% - 24\% - 19\%$
$\quad = 57\%$

Thus, 24% of the individual differences in a measured behavior is due to all of the genetic differences between people; 19% is due to environmental differences between families; and 57% is due to nonshared environmental effects.

FIG. 2.5.   Estimation of the magnitude of nonshared environmental effects e^2 using Falconer's method.

ASSUMPTIONS UNDERLYING THE TWIN METHOD

The Assumption of Equal Environments

The validity of the twin method rests on the assumption that the family environment in which MZ twins are raised is not qualitatively different from the family environment of DZ twins. This is called the *assumption of equal environments* (EEA). As shown in previous sections, the estimates of h^2_B, c^2, and e^2 are predicated on levels of genetic similarity between relatives. Estimates of genetic effect would be artificially increased if it could be shown that the similarity of MZ twins is not simply because they share 100% of their genes, but also because they are treated more similarly than DZ twins. MZ or DZ twin similarities beyond levels of genetic similarity can be caused by family members, friends, school teachers, and so on who treat twins differently from nontwins. Moreover, the similarity of MZ twins may be artificially inflated because identical twins are dressed alike more often or treated more similarly by their parents than are DZ pairs.

The EEA in most twin studies can be tested by asking twins of all zygosity groups (e.g., MZ male, MZ female, DZ male, DZ female, and DZ opposite-sex pairs) about the degree to which they were treated alike, dressed alike, placed in the same classrooms, and so on. A typical list of these questions is presented in Fig. 2.6. A statistically significant difference on any of these items would suggest that the EEA was not supported and that any estimates of genetic and environmental effect may be biased.

Fortunately, research has shown that violations of the EEA have had only a minor impact on estimates of genetic and environmental effect. For example, Borkenau, Reimann, Angleitner, and Spinath (2002) found that, although MZ twins reported being treated more similarly than DZ twins, this did not translate into increases in measured similarity in personality. Similarly, Kendler, Neale, Kessler, and Heath (1994) found that violations of the EEA had a minor correctable impact on heritability estimates for several psychiatric conditions. It is important for readers of behavioral genetic research to be aware of how a published study tests

We spend most of our time together	True or False
We attend the same school	True or False
We have the same friends	True or False
We tend to dress alike	True or False
We are in most of the same classes at school	True or False
We have always spent a lot of time together	True or False
Our parents treated us pretty much the same	True or False
We have never been apart for more than 1 month	True or False
We have almost always had the same teachers	True or False
We try to be different from one another	True or False

Have you ever been separated from your twin for more than 1 month before the age of 18? If yes, please indicate where and with whom each of you lived, what you were doing, the reason for the separation, and your age at the time.

Have you had any important experiences or training that your twin has not had? Please explain.

FIG. 2.6.   Sample questions used to assess the validity of the equal environments assumption.

whether or not the EEA holds. If a violation is reported, it is important to determine whether the reported estimates of heritability have been adjusted for its effect.

Zygosity Diagnosis

Another threat to the validity of the heritability estimate is inaccuracy in zygosity diagnosis. For example, MZ pairs misdiagnosed as DZ spuriously inflate the DZ correlation while simultaneously decreasing the MZ correlation. Heritability analyses underestimate h^2_B and overestimate c^2. The same is true when DZ pairs are misdiagnosed as MZ.

The best way to determine zygosity is to compare the similarity of DNA polymorphisms extracted from blood or buccal cells. However, the expense of DNA analysis is prohibitive. Many studies instead rely on questionnaires to assess zygosity. These questionnaires make their diagnoses based on twins' degree of physical similarity and the extent to which people of differing degrees of acquaintance confuse them. Figure 2.7 presents examples of these items. Their validity has been demonstrated by several studies that have shown questionnaires to be accurate at least 94% of the time compared to DNA analysis (e.g., Kasriel & Eaves, 1976).

The problem of zygosity misdiagnosis does not appear to concern many researchers because, if anything, they are left with a statistically conservative estimate of heritability. It is preferable to miss a possible genetic effect than to say that one is present when it is not. The latter could lead to very expensive genotyping studies that are destined to fail.

As you know, there are two kinds of twins: identical (or monozygotic) twins who have the same heredity, and fraternal (or dizygotic) twins, who only share part of the same heredity. The following questions are intended to help determine which kind you are.

1. What is the natural color of your hair? If your hair is different from that of your twin in any of the following ways, please describe these differences:
Natural color:
Rate of growth:
Hairline pattern of growth:
Thickness or texture:
Curliness:

2. What is the color of your eyes?

3. How tall are you? How much taller or shorter are you than your twin?

4. How much do you weigh? How much heavier or lighter are you than your twin?

5. If you know your blood type and Rh factor, please indicate them here.

6. As a young child, did your parents ever mistake you for your twin?
____ Yes, frequently
____ Occasionally
____ Rarely or never

7. Have your parents ever mistaken you for your twin recently?
____ Yes, frequently
____ Occasionally
____ Rarely or never

8. Have teachers ever mistaken you for your twin?
____ Yes, frequently
____ Occasionally
____ Rarely or never

9. Have close friends ever mistaken you for your twin?
____ Yes, frequently
____ Occasionally
____ Rarely or never

10. Have casual friends ever mistaken you for your twin?
____ Yes, frequently
____ Occasionally
____ Rarely or never

11. Do you and your twin look alike? Please explain.

12. If you know whether you are fraternal or identical, how do you know? How and by whom was it determined?

FIG. 2.7. Examples of questions used to diagnose zygosity.

MODEL-FITTING APPROACHES

Thus far the discussion has been focused on Falconer's method of estimating heritability (Figs. 2.3 through 2.5). A major limitation of this method is that it can only estimate h^2_B and as illustrated in Fig. 2.2, there are more genetic and environmental effects that must be accounted for. For example, broad heritability can be divided into at least two major effects: additive genetic effects and genetic dominance. To estimate them, model-fitting approaches must be used.

A *model* is an idea that has been formalized into a diagram. This diagram, called a *path diagram*, explicitly describes the hypothesized relationship between variables (e.g., *A* causes *B*) using the standard drawing methods of *path analysis* (e.g., $A \rightarrow B$). In this way, entire systems describing how variables affect and are affected by each other can be drawn. The arrows are converted to mathematical equations like those used to compute regression and correlation coefficients. Data are collected on all the variables that are then run through these equations to determine which of the hypothesized relationships are supported (e.g., the value of the arrow, also called a *parameter*, in $A \rightarrow B$ is greater than zero). If the data fit the model, the model is supported. If the data do not fit the model, the model is revised and the process repeated (e.g., trying $B \rightarrow A$). This process is called *model fitting*.

Behavioral geneticists have embraced model fitting because it is the only method that can separate additive and dominance genetic effects from h^2_B, as well as estimate c^2 and e^2 at the same time, as shown in the path diagram in Fig. 2.8. The square boxes in Fig. 2.8 represent the actual scores (e.g., scale scores from a self-report inventory or diagnosis) for each member of a twin pair. The circles represent what we cannot directly observe, in this example, the genetic and environmental factors hypothesized to influence the variability of the measured variables: additive genetic (*A*), genetic dominance (*D*), shared environmental effects (*C*), and nonshared environmental effects (*E*). The straight one-headed arrows or *paths* from the circles to the squares represent the hypothesized influence of *A*, *D*, *C*, and *E* on each of the observed variables. These paths are labeled *a, d, c,* and *e*, respectively. The values of the paths represent the strength of the relationship between *A*, *D*, *C*, and *E* on each of the observed variables and are used to compute the heritability estimates, h^2_A, h^2_d, c^2, and e^2, respectively.

The double-headed curved arrows represent the hypothesized relationship between the circles, and the values differ for MZ and DZ twins. Starting with MZ twins, the curved arrow between the additive genetic effects for each twin (between $A_{TWIN 1}$ and $A_{TWIN 2}$) would be set at 1.0 because they share 100% of their genetic material. For the same reason, the paths between the genetic dominance influences ($D_{TWIN 1}$ and $D_{TWIN 2}$) will also be set at 1.0. The path between the shared environmental effects ($C_{TWIN 1}$ and $C_{TWIN 2}$) is also set at 1.0 because, in a reared-together twin design, both members grow up in the same home. There is no path between the sources of nonshared environmental effects ($E_{TWIN 1}$ and $E_{TWIN 2}$) because, by definition, these effects are unique for each member of a pair.

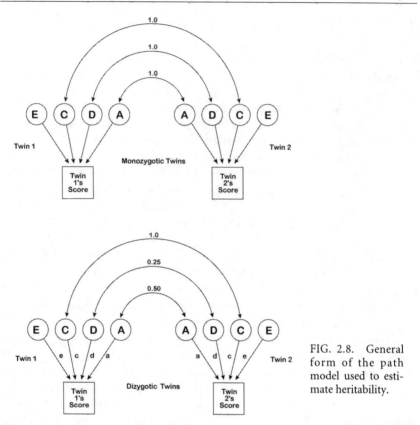

FIG. 2.8. General form of the path model used to estimate heritability.

The value of the curved arrows for DZ twin pairs is shown in the bottom half of Fig. 2.8. Fraternal twins on average share 50% of the same genetic material so the path between $A_{\text{TWIN 1}}$ and $A_{\text{TWIN 2}}$ for this group is set at .50. Genetic dominance is defined as the interaction of two genes at the same locus. Because it takes two genes to interact, a maximum of half of the total number of genes shared between DZ twins (25%) can be in a dominance relationship and common to both siblings. Thus, the double-headed arrows between $D_{\text{TWIN 1}}$ and $D_{\text{TWIN 2}}$ are set to .25. As with MZ twins, the shared environment of DZ twins is considered to be the same (remember the EEA!) and nonshared effects are unique to each member of a pair, so the path between $C_{\text{TWIN 1}}$ and $C_{\text{TWIN 2}}$ is set to 1.0 and no paths are set between $E_{\text{TWIN 1}}$ and $E_{\text{TWIN 2}}$.

There is one more theoretical consideration that must be worked into the model. It is assumed that additive genetic effects, dominance genetic effects, and shared and nonshared environmental effects are a species universal. That is, it is presumably possible to estimate these effects in all human beings, and to model this effect we assume the values of a, d, c, and e for Twin 1 to be the same in Twin 2. Furthermore, the estimates of a, d, c, and e for MZ twins must also apply to DZ twins. Thus, the model is set up so that the estimates of a, d, c, and e are applicable to all persons within the sample, regardless of zygosity.

How Models Are Fit

This section describes the process of fitting twin data into a model like that shown in Fig. 2.8. The process begins by entering into the model some values of a, d, c, and e. For example, it is commonly assumed that depression runs in families and that it is triggered by some catastrophic event. To test this hypothesis one could set the values as $a = .60$, $d = 0.0$, $c = 0.0$, and $e = .80$ to reflect the fact that additive genes are important, but nonshared environments are more important.[5] The input values usually vary between 0.0 and 1.0, and for reasons discussed later, are the square root of what one thinks the actual heritability estimate might be. In this example, if one thinks that 40% of the variance in depression is due to additive genetic factors, then the value of a would be around .63. There are other ways to reflect this hypothesis, such as $a = .40$, $d = .00$, $c = 0.30$, and $e = .70$, but one must start somewhere.

The paths with these values are traced through all of the parts of the model using the rules developed by Sewell Wright (1960) to produce estimates of the MZ and DZ correlations. These correlations are called *model-based correlations* ($r_{\text{MZ-Model Based}}$ & $r_{\text{DZ-Model Based}}$) because they reflect the conditions and values of the hypothesized model.

The next step is to compare the model-based estimates of the MZ and DZ correlations to the actual or observed values of MZ and DZ correlations computed from real data (r_{MZ} and r_{DZ}). If the model-based and observed correlations are in agreement (when $r_{\text{MZ-Model Based}} = r_{\text{MZ}}$ and $r_{\text{DZ-Model Based}} = r_{\text{DZ}}$) the model is said to provide a satisfactory fit to the observed correlations. The values of a, d, c, and e that were used to produce the values of $r_{\text{MZ-Model Based}}$ and $r_{\text{DZ-Model Based}}$ are kept as the basis for computing h^2_A, h^2_d, c^2, and e^2, respectively. If $a = .60$, $d = 0.0$, $c = 0.0$, and $e = .80$, then $h^2_A = 36\%$, $h^2_d = 0.0\%$, $c^2 = 0.0\%$, and $e^2 = 64\%$.

The degree of correspondence between model-based estimates and observed estimates is determined by taking the difference between the model-based and actual correlations and weighting it by the sample size of MZ and DZ twin pairs.[6] The resulting statistic is known to have a distribution like the chi-square statistic (χ^2) and chi-square tables can be used to test whether or not the model is statistically different from reality. Unlike most research that looks for statistical significance, the goal of model fitting is nonsignificance—that there are no significant differences between what the model produces using data and the actual data itself.

If the model and reality-based correlations do not correspond to each other at acceptable levels, the model must be modified and the whole process begins again. One

---

[5]The actual number of effects one can estimate simultaneously is limited by how many measured variables (also called *indicators*) one has data on. In the twin model shown in Fig. 2.8, there are two data points—the MZ and DZ correlations on one variable. This particular model only allows three effects to be estimated simultaneously, and the researcher is forced to decide which three. Typically, a, c, and e effects are chosen. If the researcher suspects d effects, then a, d, and e effects are selected. It is not possible with only two data points to estimate a, c, d, and e effects simultaneously.

[6]This is a very simplified description of how the results derived from the model are converted into a statistic that is compared to the observed data. Full details of the actual fitting functions and statistical tests are available in Neale and Cardon (1992).

way to modify a model is to use different values of a, d, c, and e. This could be a very tedious task as there are literally millions of different combinations of a, d, c, and e to test. Thankfully, computer programs eliminate the computational drudgery. The researcher usually begins the process by supplying start values where they think the search should begin, for example, $a = .40$, $d = .10$, $c = .10$, and $e = .50$. The choice of number might come from theory or previously published estimates of heritability.

Computers systematically test several values of a, d, c, and e in the supplied range until the model-based correlations come as close as possible to the observed correlations. This is no guarantee that the model is actually the correct one; rather, it indicates that the correlations are as close as possible within the conditions outlined in the model. The fit of the model can be very poor, as indicated by a statistically significant value of χ^2, meaning that the model must again be altered and the process repeated.

Another way to alter the model is to remove hypothesized relationships between variables. For example, the fit of the model could be improved if the path between shared environmental effects, c, and the observed variables is deleted. A model can continue to be altered in this way until a satisfactory fit is obtained. The ability to delete or add paths in a model allows the researcher to test several alternative representations of reality. At the same time, the changes in χ^2 brought about by changes in the model provide a statistically defensible means of evaluating the change, which forms the basis for model fitting and tests of the significance of additive, nonadditive, shared, and nonshared environmental effects on behavior. A typical heritability study begins this process by testing a model that specifies additive genetic (A), shared environmental (C), and nonshared environmental (E) effects. This is often referred to as an *ACE model*. The fit of the ACE model is evaluated and then the shared environmental effects are deleted from the model, turning it into an *AE model*. If this model were to provide as good a fit to the data as the ACE model, it would suggest that shared environmental effects are not significant and can be permanently left out of the model. In a heritability study, A, C, and E are alternately deleted from the model to test the significance of each. Typically, a study tests an ACE model, an AE model (which asks the question, "Are between-family effects required?"), a CE model (which asks the question, "Are genetic factors required?"), and a model specifying only E effects, to determine which best accounts for the observed twin correlations. Figure 2.9 presents a computational example of model fitting to estimate heritability.

Heritability can also vary by gender. It is not uncommon to find that the heritability of some behaviors is higher in males than in females, and vice versa. Gender differences are easily estimated by subjecting data from same-sex pairs to heritability analysis. However, these twin correlations cannot determine if different genes control the expression of a trait that is measured exactly the same way in males and females. This is accomplished by comparing the similarities of opposite-sex twin pairs to that of same-sex DZ pairs. Sex-specific genetic influences are suggested when the similarity of opposite-sex pairs is significantly less than that of male or female DZ pairs. The difference in the correlation is attributable to the gender composition of each zygosity group. When the same- and opposite-sex DZ correlations are similar, gender differences are not indicated. Behavioral genetic studies that examine the role

In this example, we fit a model estimating the magnitude of additive genetic effects (A), shared environmental effects (C), and nonshared environmental effects (E) on levels of sociability. Sociability is assessed by a ten-item self-report scale (5-point Likert format) that is summed to yield a total sociability score. The total sociability scores are subjected to heritability analysis. The scores are available on 250 MZ and 240 DZ twins raised together.

$r_{MZ} = .33$ and $r_{DZ} = .06$

Effects in the Model	χ^2	Degrees of freedom	$\chi^2_{\text{DIFFERENCE}}$	$df_{\text{DIFFERENCE}}$
Model 1: ACE	3.03	3		
Model 2: AE	3.03	4		
Model 3: CE	6.36	4		
Model 4: E	14.27	5		
Model 5: ACE vs. AE			0.0	1
Model 6: ACE vs. CE			3.33	1
Model 7: ACE vs. E			11.24	2

Model 1 hypothesizes that A, C and E effects influence sociability. Model 2 hypothesizes that C effects are zero, and only A and E effects are necessary. Model 3 is a purely environmental model, hypothesizing that no genetic effects are required and that C and E effects alone explain the aetiology of sociability. Model 4 hypothesizes that only E effects are necessary, and that individual differences in sociability are due 100% to environmental factors unique to each person in the family.

Each model has a number of degrees of freedom (df) associated with it. Usually df are based on the number of people in the study (e.g., $df = N - 1$) but in structural equation modeling it is a function of how many quantities you want to estimate from a given number of correlations (fully described in Neale & Cardon, 1992). As described in the text, the fit of the model is tested using χ^2. The critical values of χ^2 for each degree of freedom at p < .05 are:

df	Critical value
1	3.84
2	5.99
3	7.82
4	9.49
5	11.07

Thus, the χ^2 associated with models 1 and 2 is below 3.84, suggesting that they provide a satisfactory fit to the twin correlations. Model 3 is rejected because its value of χ^2 exceeds the critical value, as is Model 4.

The choice is between Model 1, specifying ACE effects, and Model 2, specifying AE effects. There is no difference in chi-square between them as shown in Model 5. To decide, we invoke the "principle of parsimony", which says that the simplest model is the one to be kept if, by all other criteria, the competing models are equally good. In this example, Model 2 wins out because it only specified two effects, A and E, as opposed to three effects in Model 1: A, C, and E. Models 6 and 7 simply confirm that they do not fit the data very well. The differences in χ^2 compared to ACE model are significant and are rejected.

The example has shown that Model 2 specifying additive genetic effects and nonshared environmental effects is all that is required to explain the MZ and DZ twin correlations. The values of "a" and "e" produced by Model 2 are .57 and .82, respectively. These values are squared $h^2_A = a^2 = (.57)^2 = .3249 \times 100\% = 32.49\%$. Similarly, $e^2 = (.82)^2 = .6724 \times 100\% = 67.24\%$.

Thus, for sociability, $h^2_A = 32.49\%$ and $e^2 = 67.24\%$.

FIG. 2.9. Estimating heritability using a model fitting approach.

of gender are generally referred to as *sex-limitation studies* because genetic effects may be limited to one gender or the other. The path models used to test sex-limited effects are described in detail in Neale and Cardon (1992).

Estimating the Heritability of Extreme Behavior

Another way of estimating heritability that has appeared in the literature is called the DeFries-Fulker method or DF method (DeFries & Fulker, 1985, 1988; Plomin, Rende, & Rutter, 1991). This method of computing heritability has become popular in studies of mental illness because it estimates the heritability of extreme-range scores as defined by the threshold liability model introduced in the chapter 1. Recall that the threshold liability model states that normal and abnormal behaviors lie on a single dimension or continuum. The model hypothesizes that abnormal behavior is the expression of disease-causing genes or exposure to critical environments whose presence in the extreme group is indicated when the estimate of h^2 is significantly different compared to the h^2 of the scores falling in the normal range.

The DF method simultaneously estimates the magnitude of genetic influences on extreme scores called the *group heritability estimate* (h^2_g) and compares it to the magnitude of genetic influences on the entire range of scores (h^2_B). A clinically significant threshold on a quantitative measure defines the distinction between normal and abnormal range scores. The hypothesis that scores from the normal and extreme ranges are influenced by common genetic factors is not supported if normal-range scores are different from the extreme-range scores (e.g., $h^2_g < h^2_B$), and vice versa. However, a finding that the magnitude of genetic influences on extreme- and normal-range scores is similar ($h^2_g = h^2_B$) suggests that the same influences underlie the entire range of scores. Note however that it is possible that qualitatively different aetiological factors influence normal- and extreme-range scores to the same degree.

The logic underlying the estimate of h^2_g is as follows: From a general population sample of twins, a proband sample of MZ and DZ twin pairs is identified (i.e., one member of a pair exceeds the clinical threshold on a continuous measure), but the score of the unaffected co-twin falls within the normal range of variation. No genetic influence on the extreme-range scores is suggested when, despite the two-fold greater genetic similarity of MZ and DZ twins, the average test scores of the unaffected MZ and DZ co-twins are equal. Genetic influences are suggested when the average unaffected MZ cotwins' test scores exceeds the average of the unaffected DZ co-twins. A test (e.g., t test) of the difference between the unaffected MZ and DZ co-twin means yields a significance test of genetic influences on the extreme scores.[7]

---

[7]For the statistically inclined, the magnitude of h^2_g was estimated with the following regression model: $C = b_1(P) + b_2(R) + A$, in which scores from the unaffected co-twin (C) are predicted by the proband score (P) and the coefficient of relationship (R: MZ = 1.0, DZ = .50) as described in DeFries and Fulker (1988). The regression weight b_1 is a measure of the average MZ-to-DZ resemblance and b_2 estimates twice the difference between the means of the MZ and DZ co-twins after covariance adjustment for any difference between the mean scores of the MZ and DZ probands. The significance of b_2 provides a test for genetic aetiology. The ratio of b_2 to the difference of the means of the total proband sample and the unaffected co-twins yields an estimate of h^2_g. A variation of this basic regression model can be used to estimate h^2_B and test whether $h^2_B = h^2_g$. However, the use of this augmented regression model is limited in that very large sample sizes are required (DeFries & Fulker) and the estimates are not constrained to be sensible (Cherny, DeFries, & Fulker, 1992).

An advantage of this analysis is that one can test multiple thresholds to help define a cutoff score on a scale that defines abnormal behavior. For example, people falling in the 60th, 70th, 80th, 90th, and 95th percentiles on a measure assessing alcohol intake (i.e., number of drinks) can be used to define the extreme group. The percentile corresponding to the point where h^2_g changes significantly could be used as the threshold to define the genetically distinct normal and abnormal groups.

THE CAUSES OF COMORBIDITY

Comorbidity is defined as "any distinct additional clinical entity that existed or that may occur during the clinical course of a patient who has the index disease under study" (Feinstein, 1970, pp. 456–457). The literature on clinical comorbidity sometimes reads like an endless cataloging of comorbid symptoms in different groups of patients. Mineka, Watson, and Clark (1998) pointed out, that as soon as this definition was applied to psychiatric disorder, difficulties delineating distinct clinical entities arose, because conditions such as general anxiety disorder were frequently comorbid with not only major depressive disorder, but also several other mood and anxiety disorders as well! Moreover, many of the same psychiatric symptoms are included in two or more diagnoses (e.g., sleep disturbances in major depressive disorder and generalized anxiety disorder) that artifactually raise the co-occurrence of disorders (Mineka et al., p. 380). They discussed several causes of this problem, from excessive splitting of diagnoses into separate disorders to methodological issues, such as the fact that higher rates of comorbidity tend to be found in studies using structured clinical interview as opposed to other methods.

A potential resolution may be possible with a determination of what causes the observed relationship between two disorders. Genetic theory hypothesizes that symptoms occur together because they are influenced by a common set of genetic or environmental factors. Behavioral geneticists index the degree to which two symptoms, disorders, or variables are influenced by the same genetic effects with the *genetic correlation coefficient* (r_G). The degree to which two variables are influenced by the same environmental effects is called the *environmental correlation* or r_E. As we learned in the previous sections of this chapter, the total genetic influence on behavior can be partitioned into the additive and dominance genetic effects indexed by r_a and r_d, respectively. Environmental effects can be split into two effects reflecting shared (r_c) and nonshared effects (r_e) that influence two or more behaviors. Figure 2.10 illustrates these effects.

On the far left of Fig. 2.10 are the severity ratings for two symptoms called X (e.g., scores on a measure of anxiety) and Y (e.g., scores on a rating of depression) collected on a sample of MZ and DZ twins. The circles represent the hypothesized additive genetic (A), shared (C), and nonshared environmental (E) influences on symptoms X and Y. The arrows from A, C, and E to symptoms X and Y represent the magnitude of each genetic and environmental effect on X and Y. These paths are the same as those used to estimate h^2_A, c^2, and e^2 described earlier.[8] Of particular interest

---

[8]The strength of the path between the genetic and environmental sources of influence on the measures is indexed simply by the square root of the heritability coefficients estimated earlier.

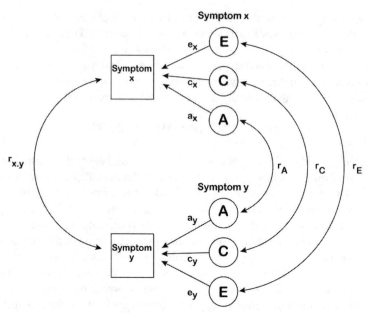

FIG. 2.10.   The relationship between phenotypic, additive genetic ($r_{x.y}$), shared (r_A), and nonshared (r_C) environmental correlations.

in this diagram is the curved line between X and Y ($r_{X.Y}$), which is the observed correlation, or comorbidity, of symptoms in the sample. The curved lines between the genetic, shared and nonshared environmental influences act on both X and Y, marked as r_A, r_C, and r_E, respectively represent the degree to which additive genetic, shared, and nonshared influences affect symptoms of both X and Y. r_A is also referred to as r_G when the particular genetic effect is not specified. Similarly, r_E refers to shared environmental influences in general. All of these correlations vary between –1.0 and +1.0. A positive correlation for r_A suggests that the genetic factors influencing X also influence Y. For example, the genes influencing the action of the serotonin transporter increase the scores on X as well as Y. A negative correlation suggests that the action of the serotonin transporter gene increases scores on X but also decreases scores on Y. On the other hand, a r_A of 0.0 indicates that the variability in X and Y symptoms comes from different genes. The relationship between the genetic and environmental correlations is summarized as:

$$r_{x.y} = (a_X \cdot a_Y \cdot r_G) + (c_X \cdot c_Y \cdot r_C) + (e_X \cdot e_Y \cdot r_E)$$

This equation states that the observed relationship between two variables is a direct function of the degree to which genetic and environmental factors independently and jointly influence each variable. Importantly, this equation opens up the possibility that a relationship may actually exist between two disorders, one that

may not be reflected in the observed correlation $r_{x,y}$. A simple example of this phenomenon is when the r_G between X and Y is high and positive, but the r_E is high and
negative. The net result on $r_{x,y}$ would be a value near zero, or quite low, suggesting
little relationship between the disorders. The reality, however, is quite different.
The two disorders are indeed related because they share a common biological and
environmental heritage.

The logic behind the estimation of r_G and r_E is much the same as that used to estimate h^2_B, c^2, and e^2. The main difference is that, instead of comparing MZ to DZ twin
similarity on a single variable, it is based on comparing MZ to DZ twin cross-correlations. The twin cross-correlation is computed by taking the first twin's score on
variable X and correlating it with the second twin's score on variable Y. Next, the
second twin's score on X is correlated with the first twin's score on Y and the two
cross-correlations are then averaged. These average twin cross-correlations are
computed on samples of MZ and DZ twins and compared. If the MZ cross-correlation exceeds the DZ cross-correlation, then a nonzero value of r_G is indicated.

Path models are used to estimate r_G in research studies because they can conve-
niently provide estimates of r_A, r_d, r_C, and r_E on two or more variables in a single model.
Figure 2.11 illustrates a path model that estimates the additive genetic correlations
(r_A) and nonshared environmental correlations (r_E) between three variables. In the
literature, readers will find that this model is frequently referred to as a "Cholesky" or

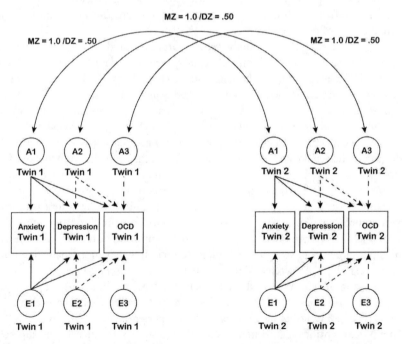

FIG. 2.11.   Cholesky or triangular decomposition model used to estimate genetic
(r_G) and environmental (r_E) correlations.

"triangular" decomposition. This method estimates how much of the genetic and environmental variance is common and unique to several variables simultaneously. For example, if the three variables were anxiety, depression, and OCD, the first genetic component (A_1) estimates how much if the additive genetic variance is common to all three; the second genetic component (A_2) estimates how much is common to depression and OCD; and, finally, the third component (A_3) estimates the genetic factors on OCD only. The same effects are estimated for the environment factors (E_1, E_2, and E_3) on anxiety, depression, and OCD. The values of these paths are standardized to provide estimates of r_G and r_E between all three disorders.

THE STRUCTURE AND ORGANIZATION OF DISORDER

The Common Pathways Model

Estimates of r_G and r_E are just the beginning. They explain why two variables are related, but do not tell us much else about the nature of disorder. For example, a question commonly asked by clinicians is, "What precisely is inherited?"; Do people actually inherit a disorder, that is, a general vulnerability to psychopathology such as major depression, or do people just inherit specific symptoms, such as moodiness, sleep disturbance, or tearfulness? To answer this question, what is needed is a sense of how symptoms are structured within a disorder. The best way to conceptualize this problem is with an example. Figure 2.12 illustrates the most common conceptualization of psychopathology.

The boxes in Fig. 2.12 contain the actual scores measured on a sample of people, such as the severity rating made on each of the symptoms of depression during a clinical interview. The variability of these symptoms is hypothesized to be a function of the presence of a unifying mental disorder called Major Depressive Episode (MDE). MDE is a theoretical construct whose presence is not directly measured, but is rather indicated by the degree to which the six symptoms appear together. What makes this drawing special is the overlay of genetic and environmental factors. In this figure, the addition of the genetic and environmental effects transforms the construct of MDE into a real entity, and these genetic and environmental effects filter down to influence the variability of each of the six measured symptoms. As such, a proportion of the genetic and environmental effects measured on each individual symptom is derived from a source that is common to all. The bottom portion of the illustration shows that this model allows for the possibility that symptoms may also be influenced by genetic and environmental factors that are unique to each. In behavioral genetic literature, the model in Fig. 2.12 is referred to as a *common pathways model*.

The common pathways model makes some statements about reality that may or may not be true. First, the model proposed suggests that the MDE construct is inherited because it has its own biological and experiential basis. This suggests that other psychic entities such as neuroticism, depression, or the id, ego, and superego may also exist and the reification of these entities in the psychological literature has been correct and is empirically defensible. Second, the observed interrelationship

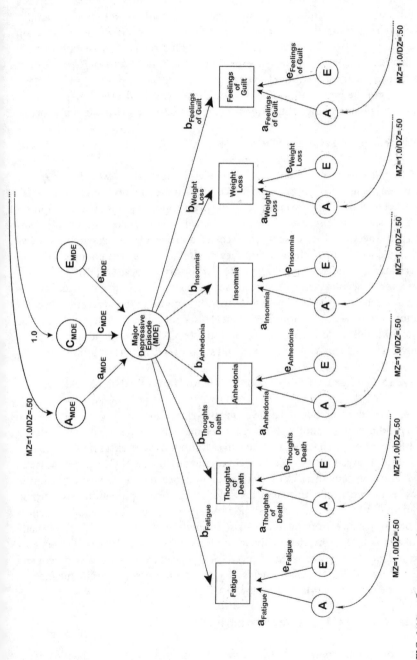

FIG. 2.12.   Common pathways model.

37

between the symptoms is due entirely to fact that each of the symptoms derives a significant proportion of its genetic influence from a common source. For example, if there is a single major gene for MDE, modifying this gene will have an impact on all of the symptoms of depression. Third, what differentiates one symptom from another is action of the genetic and experiential effects unique to each of the symptoms. The veracity of this model gives credence to the oft-used term *core pathology*. The focus of the intervention would be on the general syndrome, and genetic research and pharmacological treatments would be targeted at this general process.

The Independent Pathways Model

An alternative to the common pathways models is the *independent pathways model*, illustrated in Fig. 2.13. The main difference between the two models is that the MDE construct has been dispensed with, resulting in an important shift in how symptoms are understood and organized into recognizable psychopathologies. As in the common pathways model, the observed intercorrelation between the six symptoms is hypothesized to be due to the fact that they are influenced by common genetic and experiential factors. However, the higher order construct we call "MDE" ceases to exist as a veridical entity. Instead, MDE or any of the psychiatric diagnoses and conditions are reduced to a descriptive term that does no more than label the observed relationship between symptoms. The model does not suggest that a gene cannot be found for MDE per se, as all the symptoms still share a common aetiology. Rather, it subtly shifts the focus to the treatment and study of individual symptoms.

THE INTERPLAY OF GENES, THE ENVIRONMENT, AND EXPERIENCE

Clinicians and researchers alike have long been interested in the impact of adverse childhood events on adult behavior. For example, in the personality disorders a large body of research shows that negative childhood experiences need not necessarily lead to psychopathological outcomes in adult life (e.g., Garmezy & Masten, 1994) and to explain this lack of a 1:1 correspondence, theorists suggest that adversities in combination with genetic liabilities during development increase the risk for mental disorders. This combination of genetic and environmental influences has been formalized into the *diathesis-stress model of illness*. This model is usually invoked to explain why, despite the fact that many people may carry the genes for mental illness, or may have experienced some type of trauma, not all of them will develop mental illness. This model is very broad and does not specify the mechanisms of gene-environment interplay.

Genetic Control of Exposure to the Environment

In this form of interplay, underlying genetic factors influence the probability of exposure to adverse events (Kendler & Eaves, 1986). For example, individuals' psychopathology plays a significant role in the selection and creation of their own

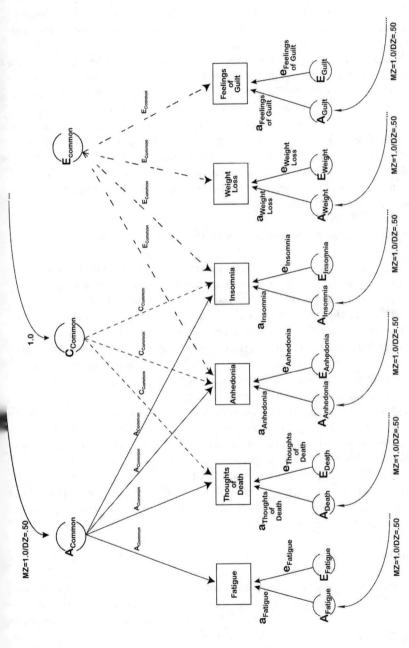

FIG. 2.13. Independent pathways model.

environment. In some fields, this phenomenon is referred to as an *amplification effect* (e.g., Paris 1994, 1996) but within behavioral genetics it is called *gene-by-environment correlation*, the extent to which individuals are exposed to environments as a function of their genetic propensities.

Three general types of gene-environment correlation have been hypothesized: *passive, active*, and *reactive* (Plomin, DeFries, & Loehlin, 1977). Passive gene-environment correlation occurs because children share heredity and environments with members of their family and can thus passively inherit environments correlated with their genetic propensities. Reactive gene-environment correlation refers to children's experiences derived from reactions of other people to the children's genetic propensities. Active gene-environment correlation is known as "niche building" or "niche picking" (Plomin, DeFries, & McClearn, 1990, p. 251). This occurs when children actively select or create environments commensurate with their underlying genetic propensities.

Environmental Moderation of Genetic and Environmental Variability

This form of interplay is also called *gene-environment interaction* (Plomin et al., 1977). One example is the effects of marriage that may either suppress or trigger the development of genetically based depressive symptoms. In addition to gene-environment interaction, behavioral geneticists discuss *environment-environment interaction* or *experience-by-environment interaction*. An example of experience-by-environmental interaction is the fact that some people can live in adverse conditions (e.g., extreme poverty) but display no ill effects because the presence of another environmental factor, such as a caring mother who attends to the emotional needs of a child, cancels out the influence of poverty.

On this note, the reader should be aware that, in most cases, genes and environment are typically assumed in common parlance to confer the liability to disorder, that is, they potentially increase the risk of developing a disorder. It is important to recognize that the interplay of genes and environment can also result in protection from the development of disorder. Within the psychiatric literature, this is often referred to as "resiliency," an important treatment factor. The concept that most children are resilient to adversity is crucial for understanding the negative impact of early adversity.

Estimating Interplay

Methods to estimate gene-environment correlations and interactions are in their infancy. The most developed are models of gene-environment interaction whose goal is to detect changes in estimates of h^2_A, c^2, and e^2 under different environmental conditions. However, actually doing this is easier said than done. One of the obstacles is that there are disagreements on how the environment should be measured. Some argue that psychosocial stressors should be measured in real time, not retrospectively. Despite the perceived advantages of real-time measurements, they are extremely difficult to obtain because they would require a well-trained army of external raters who would follow people across time from childhood to adulthood. Moreover, environmental effects can be missed if the measurement points over time are too far apart, or they can be biased if they are measured too frequently, as that would spuriously increase the salience of some stressors by continuously being emphasized.

The alternative is retrospective self-reports. The primary objection to these is that they are inaccurate for two reasons. First, ratings are subject to recall bias and do not truly reflect environmental conditions. However, research in cognitive psychology has shown that people respond to their beliefs that an event has occurred, even if it has not (e.g., Loftus & Pickrell, 1995). The most successful psychotherapies, such as cognitive-behavioral therapy, target cognitions and beliefs, so retrospective reports should not be summarily dismissed.

The second issue is that retrospective ratings can be biased by a preexisting, genetically based disorder. For example, the rating of the type and degree of parental caretaking and warmth can be attenuated by paranoia. This is a form of gene-environment correlation and shows that it can be confounded with gene-environment-interaction effects. One solution is to only use measures of the environment that are not heritable. In this way, any relationship between a person's perception and recall of an event cannot be due to a common set of pathology genes that influence both. Several twin studies of popular major measures of the environment have shown that some do not have a heritable basis (e.g., Jang, Vernon, Livesley, Stein, & Wolf, 2001). Moreover, Purcell (2002) recently proposed a method that allows for simultaneous tests of gene-environment interaction and correlation.

Apart from real-time versus retrospective ratings, a major reason for the relative dearth of gene-environment interaction research can be traced to fundamental problems in study design. The usual design is to stratify the samples into groups based on levels (usually the presence or absence) of a psychosocial stressor and to show that the heritability estimates differ for each group. However, the variable used to stratify the sample could be confounded with several other psychosocial stressors (e.g., is maternal warmth independent of maternal caretaking?), thus limiting any conclusions about the effect of the stressor to the extent that other potential moderators are adequately controlled. There is also the associated problem of sample differences. Are the samples in each strata matched for potentially competing or confounding variables such as age, sex, or socioeconomic status? More importantly, many psychosocial stressors such as levels of family conflict cannot be simply categorized as present or absent. All families experience some form of conflict that varies from low to high levels. Stratification designs simply do not lend themselves to continuously measured scales of psychosocial experience.

Fortunately, recent modifications to the path models used to estimate heritability can now incorporate continuously measured psychosocial variables (e.g., Dick, Rose, Viken, Kaprio, & Koskenvuo, 2001). One variant of this model is shown in Fig. 2.14. In this model, the psychosocial experiences reported by each twin are represented by the triangles. These can be reported levels of family con-

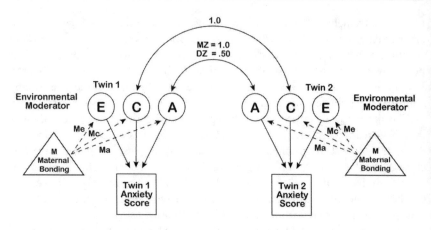

FIG. 2.14.   Gene-environment and experience-environment interaction.

flict, traumatic experiences such as sexual abuse, or levels of parental warmth. The path M_a between A_{TWIN1}, A_{TWIN2} and the psychosocial variable M index gene-environment interaction because these directly moderate the effect of genetic influences, which is converted to h^2_A. Similarly, the path M_c between the triangles and C_{TWIN1}, C_{TWIN2} indexes the degree to which the psychosocial stressors moderate the effect of shared environmental effects (c^2), and the path M_e between the triangles and E_{TWIN1}, E_{TWIN2} indexes the degree to which the psychosocial stressor moderates the effect of nonshared environmental effects (e^2). Because these methods are evolving at this time, throughout this book I discuss how gene-environment interaction and correlation effects have been tested in the context of the actual study in which they were used.

With the technical introduction now complete, the rest of the book reviews recent research in the field and discusses its implications for how mental illness is approached and understood. For many clinicians, it may appear a quantum leap to go from heritability estimates to clinical technique. The remainder of this book is designed to help the reader bridge this gap.

SUMMARY

There are two kinds of behavioral genetic methods. The first type uses DNA to identify susceptibility genes. The second group of methods is used to estimate the effect of genes, irrespective of whether they have been identified. The two most common methods of identifying the actual genes are linkage and association studies. Linkage studies are used to localize disease states to specific chromosomes. In this method, the location on a specific chromosome of genes referred to as *markers* is used as a road map for the location of possible disease genes. The marker gene may or may not be implicated in the disorder of interest, such as the genes for blood groups. The physical proximity of the disease and marker gene determines the likelihood that they will be transmitted together (i.e., are said to be *linked*) from parent to offspring. By tracing the patterns of inheritance of the marker gene and disease in a multigenerational family tree, it is possible to determine whether the disease gene is in a hypothesized location. This method has been shown to work best when disorder is caused by relatively few genes of large effect.

Contrasting with linkage methods are association methods, which determine whether specific gene forms (polymorphisms) are correlated with the variability in specific disorders or individual behaviors. Unlike linkage studies, these methods are particularly useful for testing whether genes of small effect are implicated in a disorder. Association methods require that the gene under study, called a *candidate gene*, actually be implicated in the disorder of interest. Clinical and biochemical studies are often used to select candidate genes. The genes controlling neurotransmitter function are areas under intensive investigation. In the absence of a suitable candidate, a systematic and mechanistic approach called the *genome scan* can be used to identify possible candidates. A genome scan associates a number of genes from every chromosome with disease status. The limitation of genome scans is that they require very large sample sizes of affected people and independent replications to reduce the number of false-positive results one would get by testing so many genes.

Genetic effects are estimated by comparing the observed degree of variability of a disorder in samples of family members of known genetic similarity (e.g., parents vs. children, siblings, identical vs. fraternal twins). The relative similarity, usually indexed by a correlation coefficient (r), provides an estimate of genetic effect. These methods do not just focus on genetic effect. The degree of sibling dissimilarity provides estimates of environmental effect that separate the role of the within-family environment and events from experiences, events, and conditions that are unique to each person. Estimates of genetic effect rely on the methods of path analysis, a statistical technique that allows causal statements to be made and tested (e.g., A causes B). These path analytic methods allow the interplay of genetic and environmental effects to be tested, and also test whether the relationship between measured variables is actually caused by shared genetic and environmental factors. The methods of behavioral genetics, whether the task is to find genes or to estimate their effect, are all designed to determine the role of heredity and experience on mental illness.

Chapter 3

Classification and Diagnosis

After 20 years of unparalleled advances in psychiatric research made possible in part by the DSM, researchers and clinicians have decided that the DSM doesn't carve nature at its joints.

—Steven First, cited in Helmuth (2003, p. 808)

One of the first tasks facing a clinician or clinical researcher is to describe the patient by assigning a diagnosis. Diagnoses do two very important things. First, they describe what disorder a person has and second, they impose a value judgment as to whether they are ill. Diagnostic systems are useful because they provide a common language for mental health professionals, researchers, and policy makers to discuss mental disorder. The *DSM-IV* (1994) and the World Health Organization's International Classification of Disease (*ICD*, 1992) are the best-known diagnostic systems. Both are used worldwide. There is a great deal of agreement between the systems, and each provides equivalent diagnostic codes for the other. The diagnoses contained in these systems have been developed by committees of experts to ensure that each diagnostic category fairly reflects what clinicians and experts report having observed in their patients.

Despite the care with which diagnostic systems are crafted, none are perfect because they reflect what is presently understood about a disorder and they quickly become obsolete with the publication of new research. This is reflected by the multiple editions of the *DSM* or *ICD* that appear approximately every 5 years. One of the common ways diagnoses are created and validated for each revision is by studying symptom prevalence or clusters across different populations. A diagnosis is considered valid and reliable if the same criteria are consistently found in different samples and populations. These studies establish what sets of symptoms are important in a particular disorder, but they do not address questions regarding how the symptoms are structured within a diagnosis. For example, are all of the symptoms defining a disorder equally important? Should some diagnostic criteria carry more weight than others? Another consideration not addressed by these studies is the fact that some symptoms, such as anxiety, are part of several different diagnoses. If enough symptoms are common to two different diagnoses, we are left in a quandary as to whether the person simultaneously suffers from two separate illnesses, or whether the diagnoses are inaccurate and would be improved by being amalgamated into one. This question is made more difficult by the fact that there are no guidelines for how much symptom overlap is acceptable before two diagnoses are amalgamated or conceptualized as independent entities.

One way to address this issue is to determine whether a diagnosis has an aetiological basis that is distinct from other diagnoses by demonstrating that each is associated with different loci or is caused by being exposed to specific environmental or experiential events. The presence or absence of the gene in question can be used as a criterion to define disease status. This is not the only way genetic information can be used to aid in diagnosis (see Fig. 3.1). This chapter discusses the many different ways recent behavioral genetic research has been used to classify mental disorder. The chapter begins with a review of some of the issues threatening the validity of current classification systems, then discusses some of the recent behavioral genetic research that directly addresses them. The chapter ends with two quite different suggestions for how this research can be used in the future to shape the structure of our classification systems.

FIVE LIMITATIONS OF OUR CURRENT DIAGNOSTIC SYSTEMS

Behavioral genetics researchers have addressed five broad issues that threaten the validity of current diagnostic systems: (a) the conceptualization of mental illness as a series of discrete disorders, (b) diagnostic rules that weight each symptom equally, (c) the reification of diagnoses, (d) the provision for assigning multiple diagnoses,

"'One can fantasize about replacing self-report inventories with genetic assays to assess personality traits,' says psychologist Jeff McCrae, PhD, a personality psychologist at the National Institute on Aging (NIA), 'but I doubt that will ever become a reality. The link between genes and traits is too imperfect, and we would need to discover all of the genes associated with gene-based personality assessments'. More likely—and equally important for personality researchers – is the idea that they will be able to include genetic markers among the criteria they use to validate their personality measures. '[Genetic markers] could provide one more objective indicator against which to evaluate our instrument...'" (cited in Azar, 2002, p. 13).

FIG. 3.1.   Possible uses of genetic information in psychology.

and (e) the multiaxial organization of behavior (see Fig. 3.2). The next section briefly describes each of these issues.

Mental Illness as Discrete Categories or Dimensions

A diagnosis is assigned if the patient meets a minimum number of required criteria from a prescribed set. The assignment of a diagnosis identifies the disorder and, thus automatically deems the condition as clinically significant. For example, according to the *DSM-IV* (1994, p.327), a diagnosis for Major Depressive Episode (MDE) is assigned when a patient displays either depressed mood for most of the day or diminished interest or pleasure, along with any four of the following: significant weight loss, insomnia, psychomotor agitation or retardation, fatigue or loss of energy, feelings of worthlessness and guilt, inability to concentrate, or recurrent thoughts of death. In this system, a disorder is categorized as either present or absent and there is no rating of severity. Is the depression mild, moderate, or severe? All that is known is that it is clinically significant or else the patient would not have been assigned a diagnosis in the first place. Does "clinically significant" automatically imply that the disorder is severe, or perhaps relatively mild, by just crossing over the threshold from normality? The issue of severity has been handled in a rather awkward fashion in recent editions of the *DSM* and *ICD* by providing new diagnostic categories for premorbid and less severe forms of the major disorders (e.g., dysthymia vs. depression). This approach can lead to misdiagnoses as the number of possible diagnoses increases.

Axis I: Clinical Syndromes and Disorders

Classic psychiatric disorders such as depression or complaints such as relationship problems.

Axis II: Personality Disorder and Mental Retardation

Disorders characterized primarily by long standing traits

Axis III: General Medical Conditions

Any medical disorder that might influence mental health

Axis IV: Psychosocial Problems

Includes loss of job, homelessness, and other factors that contribute to other axes

Axis V: Global Assessment of Functioning

An overall rating of the patient's social, occupational, and psychological abilities

---

FIG. 3.2.   Today's *DSM* structure. From "In Sickness or in Health?," by L. Helmuth, 2003, *Science, 303*, p. 809. Copyright 2003 by AAAS. Reprinted with permission.

The inability to rate the severity of a symptom or condition brings us to the central issues of dimensionality. A dimensional model of psychopathology states that disorder represents the extremes of the normal distribution of function. Illness is operationally defined by a threshold placed on the frequency distribution of severity. An important feature of dimensional models is that they are also multidimensional. This means that there is a frequency distribution for the severity of every symptom defining a disorder and each person is assumed to be able to display all of the symptoms to some degree. This model not only differentiates affected from unaffected individuals (depending on whether their behavior crosses a threshold), but also reflects individual differences within these groups (how people differ on each of the symptoms and combinations thereof). The quantitative nature of these models allows for statements of severity not possible in a categorical system in which people are sorted into simple "not depressed" or "depressed" categories.

It would be misleading to say that a dimensional model is the panacea to the limitations besetting current diagnostic systems. Indeed, it could very well be that some disorders are not dimensional in nature, but it behooves us to find ways to test the dimensional assumption for each of the major diagnoses. The categorical model may also unwittingly promote the idea that mental illness can be understood without reference to normal levels of function. Is it reasonable to think that depression can be studied without reference to normal variations in mood? What about social phobia without reference to shyness or obsessive-compulsive disorder with little regard to conscientiousness?

Behavioral genetic methods provide several means to investigate dimensionality. For example, computing the genetic correlation between a measure of shyness and social phobia reveals whether the normal and extreme forms of shyness are influenced by a common set of genetic liabilities. A significant correlation can be interpreted as providing support for a dimensional model, whereas a nonsignificant correlation cannot. Moreover, along with the genetic correlation, there are the environmental correlation coefficients, r_C and r_E. These can be used to provide some indication of whether a person's family life or unique experiences underlying shyness are the same as those underlying social phobia.

Are All Symptoms Created Equal?

In the previous section, the nine *DSM-IV* (1994) diagnostic criteria for MDE were listed and any five of the nine could be used to diagnose depression. This practice assumes that all nine symptoms are equally important and that each must to some extent share a common underlying aetiology. Is this a reasonable assumption? Should all symptoms be given equal weight? How would one test whether "feeling worthless and guilty" is as important as insomnia? What is the probability that "recurrent thoughts of death" and *hyperphagia* (excessive ingestion of food beyond the needed for basic energy requirements) are controlled by the same genetic and environmental mechanisms?

It is possible that each person diagnosed with depression could be suffering from quite aetiologically distinct forms of depression if each person's diagnosis was reached using a different combination of the nine criteria. The implication for genotyping studies is enormous. If all of the probands in the study were assigned the same diagnosis using different combinations of depressive criteria, the study sample may be reflecting the influence of several different (and possibly unrelated) genes, thus dooming the search for susceptibility genes from the start. One solution would be to apply multivariate genetic analyses between the criteria to understand the basis for their covariation. These analyses would provide estimates of the degree to which the symptoms shared a common genetic and environmental basis that could be used to differentially weight the importance of each symptom.

What Is Actually Inherited? The Reification of Diagnoses

A common misunderstanding about heritability estimates is that, if a genetic basis is found for a single behavior (e.g., loss of libido), it should be taken as evidence that the underlying syndrome to which it belongs is also heritable (e.g., MDE). The reverse is also assumed. If substantial heritability for the diagnosis of MDE is found, does it follow that all nine symptoms are heritable? This raises the question of what is actually inherited—the diagnosis of major depression or simply the symptoms? These two positions are illustrated in Figs. 3.3 and 3.4. If the diagnosis of major depression were the inherited entity, then the organization of the nine symptoms would resemble the drawing in Fig. 3.3 that is instantly recognizable as a common pathways model. This model postulates that all symptoms share a common aetiological basis that is derived from a central source. This model states that the diagnosis of MDE is the inherited entity and all symptoms of this disorder are simply exemplars of this higher order construct. The model also states that, if these central genetic and environmental factors did not exist, the disorder would not exist as a veridical entity.

A key extrapolation from this model is that a diagnosis made using the criteria "depressed mood for most of the day," "diminished interest or pleasure," "significant weight loss," "feelings of worthlessness," and "recurrent thoughts of death" is aetiologically the same as a diagnosis made using "insomnia or hypersomnia nearly every day," "depressed mood," "unable to concentrate," "recurrent thoughts of death," and "significant weight loss" because they are all caused by the same genes. Molecular genetic research is clearly predicated on the common pathways model.

The alternative is the independent pathways model illustrated in Fig. 3.4. This model is less restrictive because it does not require the presence of the higher order variable to which all symptoms must be related. Rather, genetic and environmental factors directly influence each symptom. In this model, there can be a single group or several groups of genes that influence some or all of the symptoms and the diagnosis as a veridical entity does not exist. In this model, the diagnosis is not the inherited entity, but rather the symptoms. A diagnosis exists as a label, a mnemonic device used to name the pleiotropic relationship that exists between symptoms.

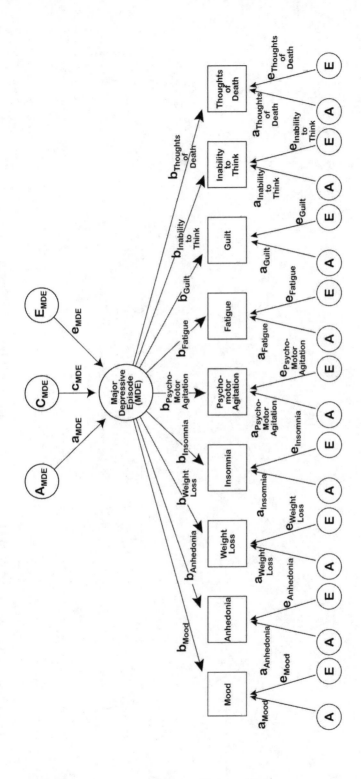

FIG. 3.3. Hypothetical common pathways model organization of *DSM-IV* (1994) MDE.

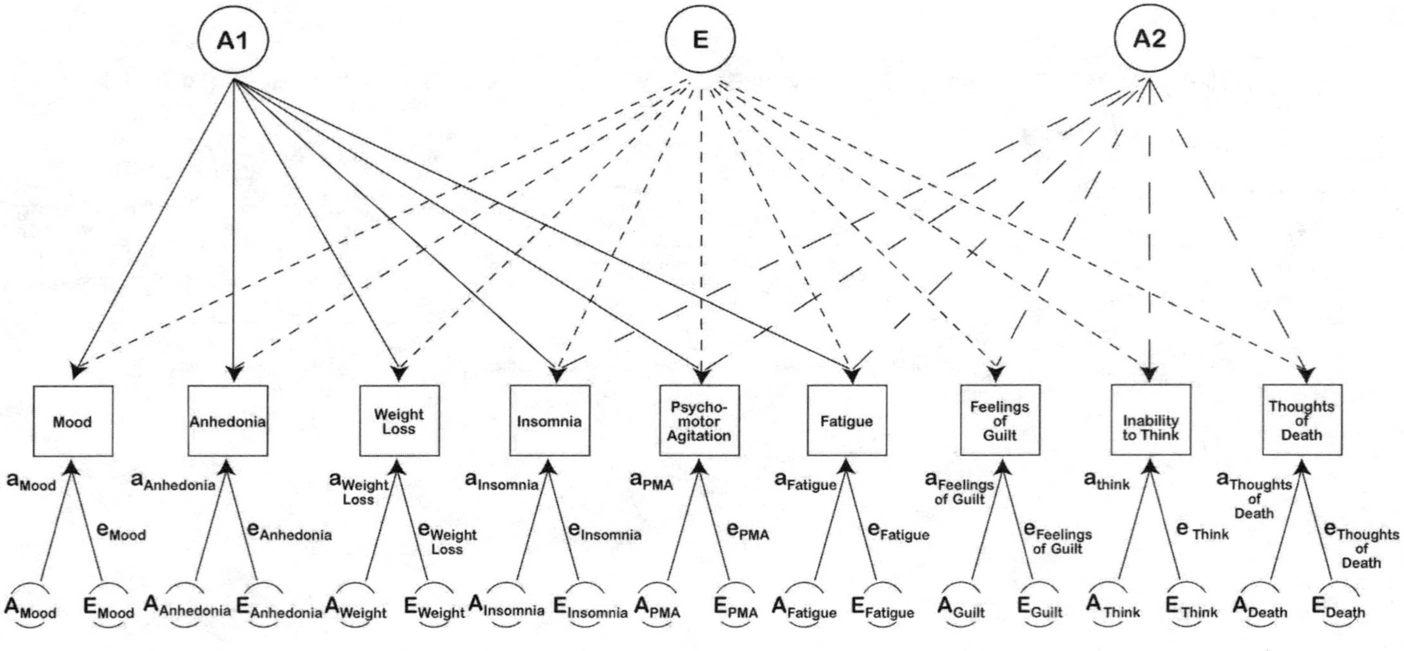

FIG. 3.4. Hypothetical independent pathways model organization of *DSM-IV* (1994) MDE criteria.

This model shifts the focus to symptoms of disorder and people are described by their symptoms rather than in terms of a disease entity.

Multiple Diagnoses

If one thing could be said for current diagnostic systems, it is that they are inclusive. The major systems have a diagnostic code to describe just about every grouping of behavior. Even if a new behavior or a new clustering of behaviors is discovered that cannot be identified with an existing code, there is always that special category "not otherwise specified" to cover it. The problem with so many diagnoses is that a single patient can be simultaneously assigned several of them, suggesting that our systems may be overly complex and contain too many separate diagnostic categories.

A concrete example of the problem is the classification of personality disorders. In the *DSM-IV* (1994), the number of personality disorder diagnoses has dropped to ten from twelve, suggesting there were too many diagnoses. Even the present ten may be too many. It is interesting to note that the ten personality disorder diagnoses have been further grouped into three clusters, reflecting shared characteristics. Cluster A includes diagnoses that reflect odd or eccentric behavior (paranoid, schizoid, and schizotypal personality disorders), Cluster B describes dramatic, emotional, and erratic behavior (antisocial, borderline, histrionic, and narcissistic personality disorders), and Cluster C reflects anxious and fearful behavior (avoidant, dependent, and obsessive-compulsive personality disorders).

One reason why diagnostic systems allow multiple diagnoses or have trouble deciding on the number of diagnoses (as with the personality disorders) may be traced to the problem of criterion overlap. Statistically, the fact diagnoses share criteria with each other can lead to increased rates of comorbidity between them. It is unclear whether the increased comorbidity is simply a statistical artifact or if the criterion overlap between diagnoses reflects the fact that two disorders are caused by a common genetic basis. The central question is whether or not co-morbidity is "noise"—a nuisance covariance that researchers should ignore or eradicate—or a "signal" indicating that current diagnostic systems are lacking in parsimony (Krueger, 1999). Multivariate behavioral genetic methods help determine the answer to this question by testing whether the observed covariation has a common biological basis. The answer will indicate if diagnoses should be amalgamated or kept separate, or if new ones should be developed to better reflect their genetic and environmental causes.

The Multiaxial System

As can be seen in Fig. 3.2, a unique feature of the *DSM-IV* (APA, 1994) is that the personality disorders are separated from the rest of the major psychopathologies. The motivation for separating them was to focus attention on the personality disorders and to reflect the fact that the personality disorders showed a more stable course compared to the other disorders. The separation has been effective in increasing their recognition in clinical settings, but it has contributed to the emergence of a new problem—the confusion of Axis I disorders with the personality disorders by both clinicians and researchers (Widiger, 2003). This results from the failure of existing criterion sets to indicate how personality disorders are to be distinguished effectively from Axis I disorders. For example, some of the behaviors used to diagnose borderline personality disorder, such as wrist slashing and purging, might be better understood as expressions of a time-limited, circumscribed mood, eating, psychotic, or dissociative disorder, rather than as maladaptive personality traits (Tyrer, 1999, cited in Widiger, 2003). Second, the boundaries of Axis I disorders have been expanding with each edition of the *DSM* to the point where evidence for the disorders as distinct clinical entities is in question. For example, what is the difference between social phobia and avoidant personality disorder? Presently, the distinction is that avoidant personality disorder is seen as a problem that relates to persons, whereas social phobia is seen largely as a problem of performance situation (Millon, 1996, cited in Widiger, 2003). The distinction is hardly convincing because a diagnosis of either can be applied to both conditions. Similarly, how is obsessive-compulsive disorder qualitatively different from obsessive-compulsive personality disorder? One solution is to determine the aetiological basis of the comorbidity between Axis I and II disorders.

THE PHENOTYPIC STRUCTURE OF COMMON MENTAL DISORDERS

The previous section outlined some of the issues threatening the validity of present-day diagnostic systems. This section reviews some recent work suggesting that the organization of the common mental disorders is quite different from the present axial structure and that the diagnoses are truly dimensional in nature (see Fig. 3.5). The data suggest that the comorbidity of ten common mental disorders can be sorted into two higher order constructs that describe disorders directed inward toward oneself as opposed to disorders that are directed outward at other people. This organization has come under intense behavioral genetic research to determine whether the relationships shown have a biological or genetic basis in an attempt to validate this structure and ultimately impact the future shape of psychiatric classification.

The organization of the common mental disorders presented in Fig. 3.5 is from Krueger's (1999) analysis of the ten most commonly diagnosed *DSM-III-R* (APA, 1987) mental disorders assessed by the U.S. National Comorbidity Survey of 8,089 U.S. civilians from 15 to 54 years old. The first factor was named "anxious misery" because it primarily accounts for the relationship between MDE, dysthymia, and generalized anxiety disorder. The second factor was labeled "fear" and describes the covariation between social phobia, simple phobia, agoraphobia, and panic disorder. The fear and anxious-misery factors are really lower order factors whose relationship was explained by a higher order factor labeled "internalizing," because together they represent disorders that are expressed primarily inward. In contrast, the covariation between alcohol dependence, drug depend-

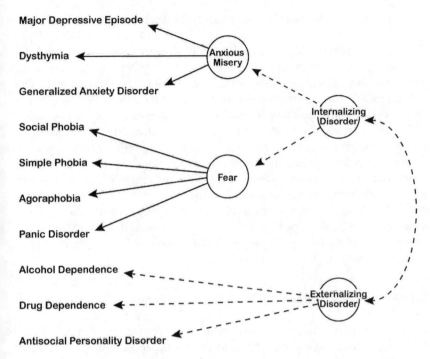

FIG. 3.5. Phenotypic structure of the common mental disorders. Adapted from "The Structure of Common Mental Disorders," by R. F. Krueger, 1999, *Archives of General Psychiatry, 56,* p. 924. Copyright 1999 by American Medical Association. Adapted with permission.

ence, and antisocial personality disorder was accounted for by a single factor labeled "externalizing" because it described maladjustment that is expressed primarily outward as antisocial, disruptive behavior. A path between internalizing and externalizing factors was also necessary to account for any comorbidity between all ten disorders.

Krueger (1999) described his model as clear evidence that common mental disorders exhibit consistently positive intercorrelations (comorbidity) that vary in magnitude (rate of comorbidity). Moreover, the patterns of comorbidity are "psychologically sensible" because they are consistent with what is observed in clinical settings. The robustness of this model was supported by Vollebergh et al. (2001), who reported finding a highly similar structure in data from the Netherlands Mental Health Survey and Incidence Study. They also found that this three-factor model was stable over a 12-month period. An immediate implication for psychiatric classification is that the axial structure of the *DSM-IV* (1994) could be modified to reflect disorders that are directed inward versus outward, in contrast to the present system where all but the personality disorders and mental retardation fall on a single axis (Krueger, McGue, & Iacono, 2001).

Behavioral Genetic Support for the Internalizing Factor

To provide support for the validity of his model, Krueger (1999) cited a number of behavioral genetic studies showing that the comorbidity between disorders stems from a common genetic basis, such as Kendler, Neale, Kessler, Heath, and Eaves' (1992b) finding that anxiety and depression were influenced in part by the same genes. For this study, clinical interviews were conducted on a population sample of 1,033 pairs of female twins for a lifetime diagnosis of *DSM-III-R* (1987) major depression and generalized anxiety disorder (GAD). The twins were divided into three groups reflecting the comorbidity of GAD and major depression and their severity. The three groups were: (a) twins with GAD for 1 month duration, (b) twins with GAD and major depression for 1 month duration, and (c) twins with GAD and major depression for a minimum of 6 months. The genetic correlations (r_G) were then computed between the three definitions to determine if they were influenced by the same genetic factors. The answer was a resounding "yes"—the values of r_G were substantial, ranging from .83 to 1.00!

Behavioral Genetic Support for the Externalizing Factor

In support of the externalizing factor, Krueger et al. (2002) assessed a sample of 421 MZ and 215 DZ pairs for alcohol dependence, drug dependence, adolescent antisocial behavior, and conduct disorder using *DSM-III-R* (1987) criteria. Antisocial personality was assessed with the "constraint" scale (specifically, a person's lack of constraint) from the Multidimensional Personality Questionnaire (MPQ: Tellegen, 1982). They fit a variety of independent and common pathways genetic models to the data and, as predicted, found that a one-factor common pathways genetic model provided the best explanation (Fig. 3.6) suggesting that the externalizing disorders are inherited as a single genetically based syndrome.

As promising as the internalizing and externalizing dimensions appear, it is important to cast a critical eye over this work. There are a number of issues that have not been addressed and it is important to highlight them at this point because they apply to any behavioral genetic study one might encounter. For instance, Krueger et al. (2002) reported that the fit of the one-factor common pathways model (Fig. 3.6) was superior to that of the other models applied to the data. However, there remains some doubt about whether this model really does provide the best explanation for the data, because their article does not indicate what other kinds of models were fitted. For example, how many alternative forms of the independent pathways model were tested? Was only a one-genetic factor independent pathways model fitted, or were others tested, such as one that specified two common genetic factors and one nonshared environmental factor? If so, did this provide a satisfactory fit to the data? One point to remember about path analysis is that the best-fitting model is only one of many possible models that can provide a satisfactory explanation of the data.

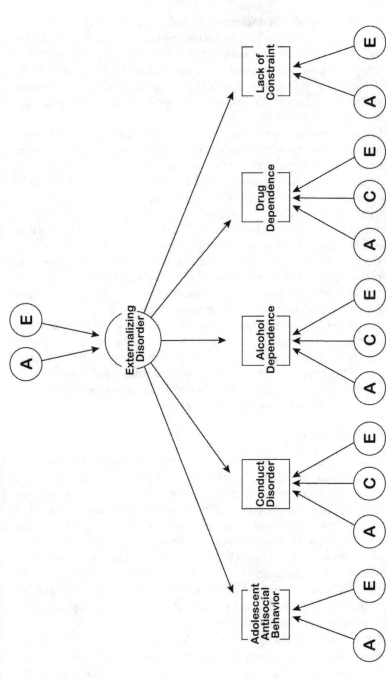

FIG. 3.6. Multivariate genetic structure of externalizing disorder. Adapted from "Etiologic Connections Among Substance Dependence, Antisocial Behavior, and Personality: Modeling the Externalizing Spectrum," by R. F. Krueger, B. M. Hicks, C. J. Patrick, S. R. Carlson, W. G. Iacono, and M. McGue, 2002, *Journal of Abnormal Psychology; 111*, p. 418. Copyright 2002 by American Psychological Association. Adapted with permission.

These doubts were confirmed recently by Kendler, Prescott, Myers, and Neale (2003), whose analysis suggests that the internalizing and externalizing factors do not exist as independent inherited entities as Krueger et al. (2002) contended. In this study, 5,600 twins were interviewed on the rate of lifetime *DSM-III-R* (1987) diagnoses for major depression, generalized anxiety disorder, adult antisocial behavior and conduct disorder, any phobia, *DSM-IV* (1994) alcohol dependence, and drug abuse or dependence.

Their first set of analyses found that an independent pathways model specifying two genetic factors, two shared environmental factors, and two nonshared environmental factors provided a good explanation for the covariance of these disorders (see Fig. 3.7). In this model, the genetic and environmental factors directly influence the covariance of the disorders and no intervening modulator variable such as "internalizing" or "externalizing" is required.

A second set of analyses was conducted on just the five internalizing disorders: major depression, generalized anxiety disorder, panic disorder, animal phobia, and situational phobia. Once again, a multiple genetic and environmental factor independent pathways model provided the most satisfactory explanation for the data (Fig. 3.8). This last set of results is interesting because it demonstrates that one set of genetic factors weighted most on major depression and generalized anxiety disorder, whereas the phobias were found to be strongest on the second genetic factor.

The pattern of the loadings in Figs. 3.7 and 3.8 supports the general idea that the internalizing disorders are organized into the anxious-misery and fear factors originally identified by Krueger (1999). However, anxious-misery and fear do not appear to be independently heritable entities, but rather are simple descriptive labels for the pleiotropic effect of genes between the diagnoses.

Criteria in Model Choice

There are occasions in which either the common or independent pathways model provides a satisfactory explanation for the data and it is appropriate at this time to discuss issues affecting model choice. A good example of the problem is Young, Stallings, Corley, Krauter, and Hewitt's (2000) genetic analysis of adolescent behavioral disinhibition. In this study, 172 MZ and 162 DZ adolescent twin pairs completed measures of substance experimentation and novelty seeking and were assessed on *DSM-IV* (1994) symptom counts for conduct disorder and attention deficit disorder (ADHD). They found that either a one-factor common pathways model (Fig. 3.9a) or a one-genetic factor independent pathway (Fig. 3.9b) provided a good fit to the data! The reported χ^2 difference between the models was a nonsignificant 1.51.

Young et al. (2000) selected the common pathways model because "[it] is a more parsimonious model than the independent pathway model and shows no significant decrement in fit by χ^2 difference test" (pp. 690–691). The dictionary definition of *parsimony* is "stingy," suggesting that they chose this model because it accounted for the data with the fewest parameters. However, parsimony is not the only crite-

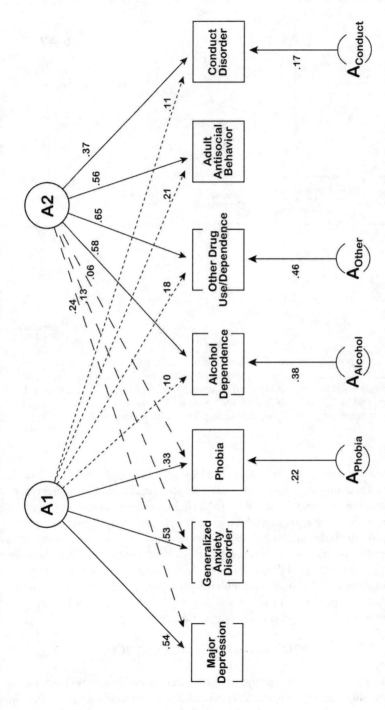

FIG. 3.7.   Multivariate genetic structure of common psychiatric disorders. From "The Structure of Genetic and Environmental Risk Factors for Common Psychiatric and Substance Use Disorders in Men and Women," by K. S. Kendler, et al., 2003, *Archives of General Psychiatry, 60*, p. 932. Copyright 2003 by American Medical Association. Adapted with permission.

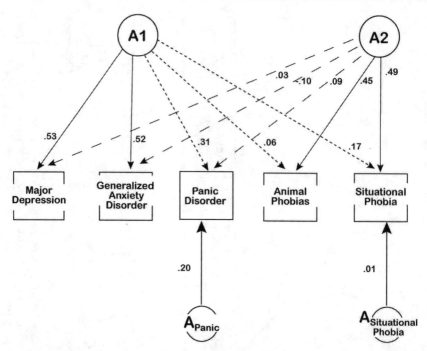

FIG. 3.8.   Multivariate genetic structure of the internalizing disorders. From "The Structure of Genetic and Environmental Risk Factors for Common Psychiatric and Substance Use Disorders in Men and Women," by K. S. Kendler, C. A. Prescott, J. Myers, and M. C. Neale, 2003, *Archives of General Psychiatry, 60,* p. 936. Copyright 2003 by American Medical Association. Reprinted with permission.

rion. Other important considerations are how stringent, rigid, and inflexible the model is. The common pathways model is more stringent because it requires that all of the lower order variables be related to the higher order ones and that all of the shared genetic and environmental influences flow through this higher order entity. In contrast, the independent pathways model does not require the presence of a higher order construct to explain genetic and environmental covariance between measures. It can be argued that omitting the higher order constructs also increases parsimony because it provides a simpler explanation for the data. In summary, when statistical guidance is lacking, the choice of model is either arbitrary, or is based on one's own theoretical preferences. Caveat emptor!

APPLYING BEHAVIORAL GENETICS

This final section examines the different ways behavioral genetic research can be used to modify current classification systems. I begin by examining an issue that the field has not really addressed—how large the relationship between disorders has to

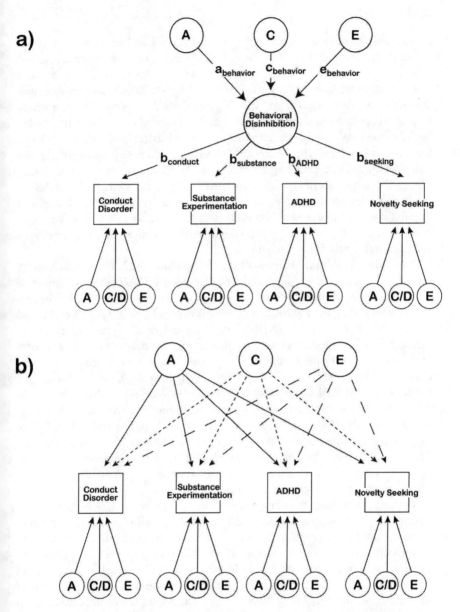

FIG. 3.9.   Two models of behavioral disinhibition. Adapted from "Genetic and Environmental Influences on Behavioral Disinhibition," by S. E. Young, M. C. Stallings, R. P. Corley, K. S. Krauter, and J. K. Hewitt, 2000, *American Journal of Medical Genetics, 96*, p. 684–695. Copyright 2000 by J. Wiley & Sons. Adapted with permission.

be (e.g., indexed by the magnitude of r_g) before the disorder loses or keeps its status as an independent diagnosis. Traditionally, statistical significance criteria (e.g., $p <$ .05) are used to guide this interpretation. However, some researchers talk about "highly statistically significant results" (e.g., when $p < .000001$) and try to draw a distinction between "significant" and "highly significant" results. This is not very helpful because statistical testing is predicated on probabilities and was designed to be "all or nothing"—either the effect happened with a degree of certainty (95% of the time) or it did not. The difference between 95% and 97% probability may not reflect a larger effect, just a larger sample size. An alternative to statistical significance is the percentage of variance accounted for. A genetic or environmental effect can be tested for significance (e.g., all estimates of h^2 and e^2 are $p < .05$), but what is important is how large the actual effect is ($h^2 = 40\%$ and $e^2 = 60\%$). However, presently there are no guidelines in behavioral genetic research regarding whether a glass of water is half full or half empty.

An example of this problem was illustrated by Wade, Bulik, Neale, and Kendler (2000), who estimated the heritability of diagnosed *DSM-III-R* (1987) anorexia nervosa and the genetic correlation between anorexia nervosa and MDE. They recruited a total of 18 MZ and 20 DZ female pairs who: (a) met *DSM-III-R* criteria for anorexia nervosa; (b) met *DSM-III-R* criteria less criterion *D* (amenorrhea); or (c) met lifetime criteria less criterion *C* (feeling fat when emaciated) to reflect severity of the condition. The heritability of anorexia nervosa was estimated at $h^2_A = 58\%$ (95% $CI = 33\%$ to 84%) and $e^2 = 42\%$ (96% $CI = 16\%$ to 68%). Within this sample, the heritability of MDE was $h^2_A = 44\%$ (95% $CI = 33\%$ to 55%) with $e^2 = 56\%$ (95% $CI = 44\%$ to 69%). The genetic correlation between anorexia nervosa and MDE was estimated at .58 (95% $CI = 36\%$ to 84%) and this translated to a finding that 34% of the genetic variability influencing MDE was in common with anorexia nervosa. They described this degree of overlap as "modest" (p. 470). However, for some researchers, accounting for less than 90% of the variance is unacceptable, whereas for others, 30% or more, such as in this paper, is quite good.

Perhaps the problem to interpreting the magnitude of effect, as in the previous example, is psychiatry's obsession with thresholds. Thresholds are defined for everything and imposes rigid, sometimes artificial black and white categories onto quantitative data whose very nature reflects shades of gray. Perhaps a better approach would be to abandon thresholds altogether and to rate the severity of all symptoms without making any judgment as to whether they fall in the "normal" or "abnormal" or "healthy" or "sick" ranges. The goal of any future classification and diagnostic system is to decide on a core set of symptoms on which all persons can be rated. An important feature of this approach is that individuals would be described in terms of their ratings on each symptom in the context of all the other symptoms (e.g., low on nervousness and all the other symptoms but high on sadness and despair), as opposed to comparing each symptom against itself (e.g., abnormally high levels of nervousness with abnormal defined by a threshold value). Classification systems would specify which symptoms would be the most informative referents for the others and this could be determined by the degree to which the symptoms share a common aetiological basis. The research in this chapter certainly supports the idea that some symptoms would be a far more informative referent than others. For example, both the phenotypic and behavioral genetic data show that disorders are related to each other in a characteristic way. Depression, dysthymia, and GAD are more related to each other than are the phobias and panic disorder, which are distinct from substance dependence and antisocial personality disorder.

However, unlike in current practice, in this symptom-focused model, there is no need to assign a label like "major depression" or "schizophrenia" for the covariance of a set of related variables or to pronounce that the person suffers from it. Dispensing with labels in this way prevents them from becoming reified and keeps the focus on the person's actual behavior. A person is not "depressed," but rather is sad and moody. A person can be very sad and moody but still be quite able to function. Illness in this model would be determined by a separate set of criteria that measures degree of interpersonal or psychosocial functioning. Do these symptoms (whatever they are) interfere with work or school? Do these symptoms affect how well the person gets along with friends, relatives, and coworkers? It is only with this final set of criteria that some kind of threshold need be imposed. In some, like ability to work, this threshold can be set by the employer with respect to productivity. In terms of interpersonal relationships, the threshold might include an assessment of how appropriately a person elicits help from others. In summary, one interpretation of the behavioral genetic research is that thresholds need not be defined for every aspect of behavior. Rather, diagnostic criteria need only describe the whole behavior of individuals without the implicit judgment of whether they are clinically ill. Illness is best determined not by the severity of symptoms, or even the presence or absence of symptoms as is done today, but is best left to a separate set of criteria that assesses the ability of the person to function.

This is one way to interpret the data, but it is not the only way. Figure 3.10 outlines a completely different interpretation of behavioral genetic research and its possible impact on diagnosis and classification. In this model, evidence of heritability for the major disorders is used to define a new axis—one that uses the presence or absence of specific genes to diagnose a disorder (Axis I). Another axis assesses whether the person has or has not been exposed to the salient environmental stressors to make a diagnosis (Axis IV). The remaining axes assess the person on cognitive abilities, neuropsychologic profiles, and so on to make a diagnosis. In short, each of the major diagnoses will be defined by whether it has a genetic basis (e.g., is linked to a specific gene); whether the patient displays specific brain-imaging profiles; whether the patient displays specific behaviors in the correct range and frequency; and whether the patient has been exposed to specific environmental or psychosocial stressors.

It should be clear that behavioral genetic research can be used in quite different ways to modify current classification systems and diagnostic practice. The ultimate form of this influence is yet to be determined. For now, behavioral genetic research

Axis I: Genotype

Genes linked to diseases, symptoms, resiliency, and drug response.

Axis II: Neurobiological Phenotype

Cognitive abilities, emotional regulation, brain imaging profile, and other qualities.

Axis III: Behavioral Phenotype

Expression of disease-related behaviors, including their range and frequency.

Axis IV: Environmental Modifiers or Precipitants

Environmental factors that alter the neurobiological or behavioral phenotype

Axis V: Therapeutic Targets and Response

FIG. 3.10.   One view of *DSM*'s future. From "Neuroscience Research Agenda to Guide Development of a Pathophysiologically Based Classification," by D. J. Charney D. et al. In: A Research Agenda for DSM-V. Kupfer, D. J., First, M. B., and Reiger D. A. (Eds.), American Psychiatric Publishing, 2002, p. 72. Reprinted with permission.

has highlighted some serious problems with current systems that will eventually force a reexamination of those systems and prevent us from naïvely accepting the comfort of the status quo.

SUMMARY

The basis for current classification schemes and diagnostic categories is based on the degree of observed relationship (comorbidity) between different disorders and symptoms. Comorbidity has become a central problem in psychopathology research because it is unclear whether it is a statistical artifact, given that the criteria used to diagnose one disorder may also belong to the set used to define other (e.g., sleep disturbances are used to diagnose MDE and generalized anxiety disorder), which artifactually raises the co-occurrence of these disorders. On the other hand, high levels of comorbidity between disorders may be an important indication that current diagnostic systems are not parsimonious enough.

Multivariate behavioral genetic research addresses this question by moving beyond the observed relationship between disorders to determine whether the relationship is caused by a common genetic basis, generically referred to as *pleiotropy*. This body of research shows that many disorders are in a pleiotropic relationship and challenges the structure of current diagnostic systems; for example, the continued separation of the personality disorders from the other disorders on a separate *DSM* diagnostic axis. The research has also suggested quite different ways to revise current diagnostic systems. One way is to revise the axial structure of the *DSM* to reflect the degree to which disorder has a genetic basis (e.g., using the presence or absence of specific genes to diagnose a disorder) and to assess whether a person has been exposed to the salient environmental stressors to make a diagnosis. Alternatively, given that virtually all disorders share a common genetic basis, it becomes meaningless to try to assign a specific diagnostic label at all. Instead, each person is rated (e.g., low, medium, high) on a set of symptoms that are found across all disorders (e.g., insomnia, sadness, anxiety), providing a direct assessment of what the person's actual problems are. Illness is defined as whether or not high or low ratings of these core behaviors interferes with a person's ability to live.

II

The Behavioral Genetics
of the Common Mental Disorders

Chapter 4

The Mood Disorders

The prevalence of depression has earned the disorder the title of the common cold of psychopathology.

—Dunn, Sham, and Hand (1993)

The mood disorders are among the most heavily researched in behavioral genetics. Heritability studies have shown that the magnitude of genetic and environmental effects varies considerably—from 0% to 70%, depending on the definition. The molecular genetic research is equally broad and varied. It has investigated a wide range of genes with mixed results: from genes known to control neurotransmitter and hormone systems to genes that have no known function.

Typically, inconsistency in results is something researchers dread. However, the variability provides the backdrop for an important theme in behavioral genetics—linking this disparity to differences in how and on whom depression was measured to address key questions about the disorder, such as: "What forms of depression are heritable?" Are specific symptoms differentially heritable? Is a general liability to depression inherited? Is depression in females the same as in males? What is the relationship between different forms of depression, such as bipolar and unipolar? The outcome of the molecular and behavioral genetic research on these questions has resulted in a shift in the understanding of depression from a broad and monolithic disorder to a collection of individual symptoms that vary in severity and aetiology. The notion that depression may not be inherited as a unitary disorder is highlighted by the frequently contradictory results from molecular genetic studies.

IDENTIFYING SUSCEPTIBILITY GENES FOR DEPRESSION

Neurotransmitter Studies

The serotoninergic system has received a great deal of attention because clinical studies have shown that transport of this neurotransmitter is significantly lower in patients diagnosed with major depressive disorder (MDD or "unipolar depression"; see also Cowen, 1993, for a review). Serotonin has also been implicated in related forms of depression, such as seasonal affective disorder (SAD). For example, positron emission tomography (PET) studies have shown reduced levels of the serotonin transporter and low production of tryptophan hydroxylase, an amino acid precursor of the synthesis of serotonin in SAD patients (e.g., Willeit et al., 2000).

The gene that controls the transport of serotonin is the serotonin transporter repeat-length polymorphism, or 5-HTTLPR, gene. The gene comes in either a short (s) or a long (l) form. Each parent contributes one of these genes that would yield one of three possible genotypes: s/s, l/l, or s/l. Early association studies suggested that the short form of the allele was the putative disease gene. For example, Collier, Arranz, Sham, and Battersby (1996) showed that frequency of genotypes containing the short form of the gene was elevated in a large sample of 454 patients diagnosed with bipolar or unipolar depression, compared to 570 healthy controls. However, this elevation in scores was not quite statistically significant. Recently, Geijer et al. (2000) replicated this lack of association. They did not find any differences in the frequency of 5-HTTPLR polymorphisms in suicide attempters diagnosed with unipolar depression compared to healthy normal controls. They also found no differences in the gene frequencies for the serotonin receptor 2A or the tryptophan hydroxylase gene.

Rosenthal et al. (1998) reported that the frequency of the short allele was higher (44.8%) in a sample of 97 patients with SAD compared to a sample of 71 healthy controls (32.4%). This is important because SAD is defined as a variant of recurrent MDD whose essential feature is the onset and remission of major depressive episodes at characteristic times of the year (*DSM-IV*, 1994). Unfortunately, several studies have failed to replicate the association. Lenzinger et al. (1999) carefully matched 18 drug-naïve (people who have not received medication for their condition) SAD patients with healthy controls and found no association. This finding was also replicated using samples drawn from Sweden, Finland, and Germany (Johansson et al., 2001).

The frustration that characterizes research on serotonin also applies to the research on the other major neurotransmitters. Neither the genes controlling the transport nor those controlling the reception of dopamine have been consistently associated with bipolar depression (e.g., Byerley, Hoff, Holik, & Coon, 1994; Holmes, Brynjolfsson, Brett, & Curtis, 1991; Serretti et al., 1999). Similarly, few significant associations between the peripheral benzodiazapine receptor gene and bipolar or other depressive disorders (e.g., Kurumaji, Nomoto, Yamada, Yoshikawa,

& Toru, 2001) or differences in monoamine oxidase gene variants (e.g., Syagailo et al., 2001) have been found.

Hormones, Proteins, and Depression

Another strategy has been to examine other biochemical systems for possible candidates. Recent research on age-related changes in hormone systems has yielded some positive associations worth investigating. Seidman, Araujo, Roose, and McKinlay (2001) focused on the androgen receptor gene because of clinical findings that depressive symptomology increases as levels of age-related testosterone levels decrease. In a sample of 1,000 men, 110 were classified as depressed using a cutoff score on the Center for Epidemiologic Studies Depression Scale (CES-D: Radloff, 1977), a popular self-report scale of depressive symptomology. All subjects had testosterone levels measured and were genotyped for the repeat length of the CAG gene, a marker associated with androgen receptor function. They found that depressive symptomology was significantly and inversely associated with total testosterone levels in men with shorter CAG repeat lengths, but not in men with moderate and longer repeat lengths.

Another age-related target of research is the Apolipoprotein-E e4 allele (APOE). Although this gene is best known as a risk marker for Alzheimer's disease, it is thought to be important in depression because depression is one of the diagnostic criteria for dementia. Several positive associations have been reported between the APOE allele and late-onset depression (e.g., Steffens et al., 1997). More recently, Stewart, Russ, and Richards (2001) found that the APOE allele was present in 69% of subjects who display subjective memory impairments with depression, as opposed to only 28% of subjects with either depression or impairments in subjective memory. Despite these positive associations, Mauricio et al. (2000) found no association between the APOE allele and changes in depression scores in a sample of 113 seniors who were followed longitudinally for 5 years.

Other genes under active study are those that mediate the immune system response (e.g., activity of natural killer cells, antibody production, T-cell activation) and that are suspected to differ between patients diagnosed with major depression and other populations (see Maes, Meltzer, Scharpe, & Bosmans, 1993, for a review). On a more positive note, a research trend producing fascinating and clinically relevant results does not search for depression genes per se, but rather genes that control the effects of antidepressants. A good example of this research is the work on the genes that control liver enzymes and how they metabolize medication (e.g., Murphy, Kremer, Rodrigues, & Schatzberg, 2003). Another interesting twist is the report of significant associations between depression and genes that have no known function. For example, Zubenko, Hughes, and Stiffler (2002) found that the frequency of the gene D2S2944—found on the long arm of chromosome 2—was about three times higher in the female patients diagnosed with *DSM-III-R* (1987) recurrent early-onset major depressive disorder (MDD) compared to healthy female controls. In contrast, no increase in the frequency of the D2S2944 gene was found in males with this disorder, suggesting that a major sex difference exists in the aetiology of early onset MDD.

At this time, some of the most consistent molecular genetic results have come from linkage studies. Recent reviews of bipolar depression have noted several significant linkages on chromosome 18p (see Gershon et al., 1998). Chromosome 18 is of interest for another reason: several linkages to schizophrenia have been reported on this chromosome (see Gershon, 2000) and both disorders (bipolar depression and schizophrenia) have also been linked to chromosome 13q (Blouin et al., 1998; Detera-Wadleigh et al., 1999). These linkage studies suggest that what is inherited is not a specific disorder, but rather a general liability to psychopathology. Gershon (2000) refered to these as "nonspecific psychopathology genes"—genes that are shared by families but do not coaggregate in families. It is unclear at this time what this general vulnerability to psychopathology might be, but if these genes exist, their identification would help us to understand the biology of susceptibility, develop new diagnostic tests for this vulnerability, and focus attention on the genetic and environmental factors that differentiate various manifestations of disorder.

In summary, the most recent molecular genetic results remain as inconsistent as earlier research. Thus, Kendler, Neale, Kessler, Heath, and Eaves' (1992a) comment that "in the absence of replicated positive results of linkage analysis, twin and adoption studies provide our only method for disentangling the genetic and non-genetic sources of familial resemblance for depression" (p. 257) is as valid today as it was a decade ago. The next section examines this now very large body of research.

THE HERITABILITY OF UNIPOLAR DEPRESSION

Female Depression

Heritability studies worldwide have shown that genetic factors account for between 30% and 40% of the total variation in MDD among general population females. In the United States, Kendler et al. (1992a) estimated the heritability of *DSM-III-R* MDD in a sample of 1,033 female twin pairs from the United States at 42%, with the remaining 58% due to nonshared environmental (e^2) factors. More recently, Kendler and Prescott (1999a) reported the heritability of MDD at 39% using a sample of 3,790 female twin pairs from Virginia. Shared environmental (c^2) effects were again estimated at zero, with the remaining 61% attributable to nonshared environmental effects.

These estimates were replicated in a large community-based sample of twins from Australia. Bierut et al. (1999) estimated the heritability of *DSM-III-R* (1987) MDD at 44% (95% CI: 29–53%). When the newer *DSM-IV* (1994) criteria were applied, the heritability estimate remained much the same at 36% (95% CI: 15%–46%). Heath et al. (1999) reported similar results: Additive genetic effects accounted for 26% of the variability in *DSM-III-R* MDD and 44% in *DSM-IV* MDD. To underscore the stability of these results across countries, a recent meta-analysis of family and twin studies worldwide estimated that 37% (95% CI: 31%–42%) of the variability in female MDD was attributable to genetic influences (Sullivan, Neale, & Kendler, 2000).

Male Depression

In contrast, the heritability of depression in males is noticeably lower. Among Australian male pairs, Bierut et al. (1999) estimated the heritability of male *DSM-III-R* (1987) depression at 24% (95% CI: 0.00%–39%). This estimate dropped a bit lower to 18% (95% CI: 0.00%–26%) when current *DSM-IV* (1994) criteria were applied. A significant aspect of these findings is that the lower boundary of the 95% confidence interval includes zero, suggesting that male depression may not be heritable at all. This was demonstrated when the definition of depression was modified to reflect severe depression. Among males, heritability dropped to a mere 1% (95% CI: 0.00%–60%), but remained high at 38% (95% CI: 0.00%–52%) among females.

The question of gender differences was examined in further detail by Kendler and Prescott (1999a). They first estimated the heritability of depression in males and females. They found h^2_A = 39% for each gender, which is inconsistent with reports from other studies. However, it can be argued that this is not the case because the estimates fall within reported confidence intervals from other studies. Nevertheless, the important point here is that it is commonly assumed that the causes of depression in males are not much different from the causes of depression in females. The similarity of the magnitude of male and female heritability in this study is consistent with this assumption, but remains to be tested by estimating the genetic correlation (r_G) between male and female depression. The r_G was far from unity (1.0), being estimated at 0.57, indicating that a significant proportion of the genetic factors underlying male and female depression are not shared, and that the route to depression is gender specific.

Heritability Based on Revised Diagnostic Criteria

The research just summarized is based entirely on standard diagnostic criteria. As outlined in chapter 3, this is problematic because this system weights all symptoms equally and yields patient groups composed of different combinations of symptoms. Each patient thus presents with quite different forms of depression that could be caused by diverse genetic and environmental causes. This problem is exacerbated by the fact that diagnostic systems force behavioral phenomena into categories that deem the disorder present or absent without indication of actual severity.

A popular solution has been to revise the definitions to better reflect differences in severity. Two such systems, the Washington University criteria (WUC: Feighner, Robins, & Guze, 1972), and the Research Diagnostic Criteria (RDC: Spitzer, Endicott, & Robins, 1978) are commonly used across North America in clinical and research settings. The WUC and RDC criteria are frequently employed in conjunction with *DSM-III* (1980), *DSM-III-R* (1987), and *DSM-IV* (1994) criteria. Superficially, these definitions of depression are quite similar.

They all specify periods of dysphoric mood or pervasive loss of interest or pleasure. The RDC is the most similar to the *DSM* system in that a diagnosis of depression requires that a patient meet a minimum five out of nine criteria. However, the RDC assesses more severe forms of depression because it requires that the duration of dysphoric features last at least 1 week and that the person sought or was referred to help from someone during the dysphoric period, took medication, or had impairment with family, at school, at work, or socially. The WUC criteria are the most different. Only the WUC was designed at the outset to allow differential diagnoses of "definite" or "probable" depression. The original RDC definitions have been modified to include these subtypes. The difference between definite and probable depression is in the number of criteria. Definite depression requires the patient to meet five of eight criteria, whereas probable depression requires only four of eight criteria. The WUC criteria assesses the most severe forms of depression because a diagnosis cannot be made unless the illness lasts at least 1 month (4 weeks) with no prior existing psychiatric criteria.

By estimating the heritability of different subtypes, it is possible to determine whether more severe forms or particular sets of symptoms are differentially heritable. Figure 4.1 presents the heritability of nine different definitions of major depression reported by Kendler et al. (1992a) on females. In general, the estimates are very similar, ranging between 24% and 39%, with no c^2 effects.

In contrast, quite dramatic changes in male h^2 are seen with more severe forms of depression. Lyons et al. (1998) estimated the heritability of *DSM-III-R* (1987) MDD at 36% (95% CI: 25%–47%) using a sample of 3,372 male pairs who were vet-

Definition of Depression	h^2_A
DSM-III (1980)	.39
DSM-III-R (1987)	.42
RDC definite	.44
RDC probable	.39
Gershon	.45
WUC primary and secondary probable	.33
WUC primary, secondary, definite	.33
WUC primary, probable	.21
WUC primary, definite	.24

FIG. 4.1.   Heritability of major depression in women. Adapted from "A Population-Based Twin Study of Major Depression in Women," by K. S. Kendler, M. C. Neale, R. C. Kessler, A. Heath, and L. J. Eaves, 1992, *Archives of General Psychiatry, 49,* p. 261. Copyright 1992 by American Psychiatric Publishing, Inc. Adapted with permission. RDC = Research Diagnostic Criteria; WUC = Washington University Criteria; Gershon = modified RDC criteria from Mazure and Gershon (1979).

erans of the Vietnam War. However, this estimate dropped to zero when the diagnostic criteria were modified to reflect dysthymia, mild and moderate depression—the kinds of depression that are typically found in general population samples. When the criteria were modified again to reflect severe or psychotic depression, h^2_A jumped back up to 39% (95% CI: 20%–56%).

The studies reviewed here converge to show that the heritable basis of MDD in women ranges from 20% to 40%. Among males, the influence of genetic effects is somewhat lower, with only the most severe forms having a significant genetic basis and being specific to each gender. In general, these estimates do not seem particularly high and are at odds with the beliefs held by many clinicians and researchers that genetic influences are much greater. Certainly, many molecular genetic studies are predicated on this belief. As a result, many have asked whether heritability studies of depression have underestimated genetic effects.

Has Heritability Been Underestimated?

How might the heritability of depression have been underestimated? One of the obvious culprits is the systematic error inherent in the way psychopathology is measured. For example, many twin studies of psychiatric disorder administer psychiatric interviews not in person but over the telephone, where subtle but important signs (e.g., body language, response styles) can be missed. To investigate this possibility, Kendler, Neale, Kessler, Heath, and Eaves (1993) collected data on the lifetime history of major depression on a sample of 721 female twin pairs drawn from the general population, first using a self-report questionnaire and then again by personal interview. Initial analyses showed that agreement between personal interview and self-report was quite modest: Test-retest reliability was estimated at a dismal k = .34. or "kappa" is interpreted like a correlation coefficient. A value of 1.0 indicates perfect agreement and zero indicates no agreement between assessments, raters, or any other measurement tool.

To correct for this lack of agreement, a multiple regression analysis was used to select a combination of variables from self-reports and personal interviews that yields a highly reliable "index of caseness." Kendler et al. (1993) found that the most reliable indices of depression were: (a) number of depressive symptoms, (b) treatment seeking, (c) number of episodes, and (d) degree of impairment. When these criteria were used to assess and diagnose depression, additive genetic factors jumped to account for a whopping 70%!

McGuffin, Katz, Watkins, and Rutherford (1996) found similar results. Their sample consisted of 177 twin pairs in which at least one member was diagnosed with unipolar depression using DSM-IV (1994) criteria from UK hospital admissions. In this study agreement among raters was exceptionally high with k = .92. The MZ twin concordance rates for male, female, and the total sample were 45.8%, 45.5%, and 45.6% respectively, which is more than double the DZ concordance rates of 14.8%, 22.0%, and 20.2%. From these data, heritability was estimated at 75%.

An interesting aspect of this study is that the greatest MZ to DZ concordance ratio occurred when: (a) the duration of the longest episode was less than 13 months, (b) there were multiple episodes, and (c) most uniquely, the symptoms represented an "endogenous" rather than "neurotic" pattern. The distinction between neurotic and endogenous depression comes from the ICD-9 (1994) diagnostic system. Neurotic depression is described as depression that occurs as a result of a distressing experience (e.g., loss of a cherished person or possession) and is characterized by the presence of anxiety. In contrast, endogenous depression is characterized by a lesser degree of anxiety and there is no clearly recognizable event that may have precipitated onset. It is also described as a widespread mood of gloom and wretchedness, reduced activity, and possible restlessness and agitation and also is recognized as having a marked tendency to recur.

The Heritability of Depressive Symptoms

The finding that endogenous and neurotic patterns of depressive symptoms may be differentially heritable is a key finding because it indicates that some aspects of depression might be under greater genetic control than others. The finding directly challenges the assumption underlying current diagnostic systems that all symptoms are created equal and can be used interchangeably.

Which symptoms are heritable and which are not was examined by Jang, Livesley, Vernon, Taylor, and Moon (2004), who jointly analyzed the items from three popular self-report measures of depressive symptomology: the Beck Depression Inventory (BDI: Beck & Steer, 1993), the Center for Epidemiologic Studies Depression Scale (CES-D: Radloff, 1977), and from the revised Symptom Check List (SCL-90-R: Derogatis, 1994), three items measuring sleep problems, Depression, Anxiety, Phobic Anxiety, and Somatization subscales. Together these scales cover a broad range of cognitive, affective, behavioral, and somatic symptoms of depression.

The measures were completed by 336 general population twin pairs. All of the items were subjected to factor analysis that yielded 14 independent factors of depressive symptoms. Heritability analysis showed that only seven factors had a heritable basis: insomnia/hypersomnia (35%), loss of libido/pleasure (22%), positive affect (18%), loss of appetite (20%), feelings of guilt and hopelessness (30%), suicidal thoughts (18%), and physical symptoms of anxiousness (20%). All of the variability on the remaining factors including feelings of loneliness, phobias, backaches and pains, crying, interpersonal problems, nausea and headaches, and psychomotor retardation could be accounted for entirely by c^2 and e^2 effects.

These analyses suggest that somatic symptoms such as loss of appetite or libido, or symptoms that reflect items found on a personality questionnaire (e.g., feelings of guilt and hopelessness; positive affect) are heritable. The remaining symptoms appear to reflect cognitive and somatic responses to negative life events and experiences. These symptoms are best described as "reactive" (similar to "neurotic depression" described in McGuffin et al., 1996) in that they are triggered by psychosocial stress.

One possible explanation for the differential heritability of depressive symptoms is that each reflects differential sensitivity of specific brain areas to biochemical versus nonbiochemical interventions. A number of neuroimaging studies suggest this intriguing possibility. For example, Martin, Martin, Rai, Richardson, and Royall (2001) showed that different types of treatment for depression result in functional changes in blood flow in the brain. The study subjects were 28 adult males and females who had had a *DSM-IV* (1994) major depressive episode, a Hamilton Depression Rating Scale (HAM-D: Hamilton, 1967) score of 18 or higher, and had not been taking antidepressant medication for at least 6 months.

Thirteen of the patients received up to sixteen weekly 1-hour sessions of interpersonal psychotherapy (IPT). IPT is a time-limited technique that helps patients understand their low mood in terms of complicated bereavement, role transition, role dispute, or interpersonal deficits. The patient is taught strategies to change and adapt to interpersonal problems. The remaining fifteen subjects received 37.5mg venlafaxine hydrochloride twice daily. Both treatment groups improved substantially and all patients were imaged at 6-week intervals.

The image-mapping results were startling. The venlafaxine hydrochloride group showed greater right posterior temporal and right basal ganglia activation, whereas the IPT group had right limbic posterior cingulate and right basal ganglia activation. Only IPT caused limbic blood flow, but both IPT and venlafaxine groups had increased blood flow in the basal ganglia. There is another body of research suggesting that cingulate function—in particular the so-called "area 24a" (e.g., Mayberg et al., 1997)—is more sensitive to pharmaceutical intervention than other areas.

ENVIRONMENTAL AND PSYCHOSOCIAL FACTORS IN DEPRESSION

Clinical research shows that many depressive episodes are often precipitated by some monumental event in a person's life. This section explores the salient environmental factors that have been identified and the role they play in the onset and maintenance of depressive symptoms. One of the first studies to identify the environmental risk factors for MDD was that of Kendler, Kessler, Neale, Heath, and Eaves (1993). They simultaneously examined environmental and genetic risk factors in a sample of 680 female general population twin pairs who were interviewed on an extensive battery of questions assessing environmental conditions and experiences at three consecutive 13-month intervals.

The environmental factors assessed were: (a) parental warmth; (b) lifetime trauma such as sexual assault, physical assault, or life-threatening accidents or illness; (c) actual and perceived levels of social support and integration (e.g., perceived support of friends and relatives, frequency of contact with friends and relatives, frequency of attendance at clubs or organizations, religious attendance); and (d) presence of a confidant. They were also assessed for a history of previous major depression (three of the following for at least a 2-week duration: depressed mood, appetite disturbance, decreased energy, feelings of worthlessness, difficulties in concentrating). In addition, they were assessed on the person-ality trait of neuroticism.

At the second testing session they were interviewed for major depression in the last year in addition to loss of a parent (separation from biological mother or father before age 17 not as a result of military service, business travel, etc.). They were also asked about any recent difficulties or stressful life events in the past year—assault (assault, rape, or mugging); divorce or separation (divorce, marital separation, bro-ken engagement, or breakup of other romantic relationship); major financial prob-lems; serious housing problems; serious illness or injury; job loss (laid off from a job or fired); legal problems (trouble with police or other legal trouble); loss of confi-dant (separation from other loved one or close friend); serious marital problems; robbery; and serious difficulties at work.

Approximately 17 months later, the women received a final psychiatric inter-view for MDD and stressful life events in the last year. Analyses showed that the strongest predictors were, in descending order: (a) stressful life events in the past year, (b) genetic factors, (c) previous history of major depression, and (d) the per-sonality trait of neuroticism. They also found that 40% of the heritable influences on depression were mediated by: (a) prior history of depressive episodes, (b) num-ber of stressful life events, (c) lifetime traumas, and (d) trait neuroticism, clearly in-dicating that gene-environment interplay is important in the liability of MDD and accounting for the variability of heritability estimates presented earlier. In total, all of the predictors together accounted for 50.1% of the total variance for liability to depression.

The Kendler, Neale, Kessler, Heath, and Eaves (1993) study highlighted the im-portance of stressful life events as a predictor of MDD. It is interesting to note that other factors typically thought to be very important, such as lack of social support, did not emerge as predictors but it is possible they were overlooked because of how they were assessed. Brown (1998) noted that behavioral genetics researchers tend to use broad measures of environmental conditions that are little more than faceless aggregated counts of events. He also noted that environmental events that are pre-dictive of different disorders are often combined into a single measure. An example he gave is that "loss" events shown to be predictive of depression and "danger" events shown to be predictive of anxiety disorders are often combined into a single measure. He wrote that the concept of loss is a detailed one, including not only loss of a person, but loss of role, resources, or a cherished idea about oneself or someone close. However, behavioral genetics researchers tend to treat all types of loss as in-terchangeable when, in fact, some kinds of loss may have more of an impact on de-pression than others.

Another issue is the degree to which the occurrence of a stressful life event "matches" or is congruent with an ongoing difficulty. A mother learning that her son was arrested for drug dealing would be said to match with his long-standing de-linquent and irresponsible behavior (Brown, 1998, p. 366). In this example, the stressful life event—the arrest of a child—will have less impact on the mother if it is congruent with the child's behavior because she would have, in a sense, expected it to occur. Conversely, the impact of this event on the mother would be greater if it was not congruent with the child's characteristic way of behaving. Brown also noted that many of the environmental questionnaires used in behavioral genetic studies are self-reports that are described as "objective" measures of events and experiences. He raised the possibility that genetically based personality features can influence, for example, the frequency of questionnaire item endorsement. As a result, the responses may not accurately reflect the normal frequency of events. For example, "In a ghetto population ... more adventurous, novelty seeking children (dispositions probably partly genetically determined) may spend more time on the streets and thereby be more likely to witness a drug related murder" (Brown, p. 369). He referred to this as "event-proneness" or, in the parlance of behavioral genetics, gene-environment correlation that is often not tested for.

Despite Brown's (1998) spin on the issue, it would be shortsighted to understand event-proneness as a methodological problem. It must be remembered that quantitative genetic theory predicts that genetically moderated effects on an environmental circumstance or condition can have a potentially greater impact than the direct effect of the circumstance itself. The message is that deliberate attempts at obtaining only objective assessments of the environment may be a limited strategy. The key for researchers is not to try to eliminate these effects, but to study them in their own right.

Gene-Environment Interplay

Gene-Environment Correlation. On that note, I now turn to the literature examining gene-environment correlation. I must digress for a moment to specify how the term *gene-environment correlation* is used. In recent years this term has been used in two different ways. The theoretical usage of the term describes the phenomenon of genetic mediation of the environment, illustrated by Brown's (1998) example of event-proneness. Another example of event-proneness is when a parent notes that their child has natural musical ability while banging spoons on a pot and as a result provides music lessons and a piano. The joint occurrence of the spontaneous onset of musical ability (the gene) and the piano and lessons (the environment) is a form of gene-environment correlation (specifically, the reactive type described in chapter 2). The other use of the term is in an applied context—specifically, the genetic correlation (r_G) between a measure of the environment (which has some heritable aspects) and another heritable variable whose genes are thought to influence how the environment is perceived (e.g., depression, personality, etc.) as described below. It is important that the reader of behavior genetics papers distinguish between the two.

Kendler and Karkowski-Shuman (1997) tested whether genetic risk factors for MDD increased the risk of experiencing a significant life event. A sample of 938 pairs of adult female twins was assessed twice (17 months apart) on significant life events (similar to those used in the Kendler, Neale, Kessler, Heath, & Eaves [1993] article described earlier) and a unique class of variables labeled "network variables."

Network variables are events that happen primarily to, or in interaction with, an individual in the respondent's social network. These items included death or severe illness, and interpersonal problems with a spouse, friend, coworker, child, or parent that were combined into three categories: (a) death in network, (b) illness in network, and (c) trouble (getting along) with network.

Kendler and Karkowski-Shuman (1997) first tested each of the environmental variables to determine if they had a heritable basis. They found that: (a) serious marital problems, (b) divorce or breakup, (c) job loss, (d) serious illness, (e) major financial problems, and (f) trouble getting along with others in the network all had a significant heritable basis. When the genetic correlations between these variables and MDD were estimated they found significant associations with divorce or breakup ($r_G = 1.00$), serious illness ($r_G = .53$), and major financial problems ($r_G = .41$). Although these genetic correlations appear large, only between 10% and 15% of the impact of genes on the risk for major depression is mediated through significant life events—"an amount that is neither trivial nor overwhelming" (Kendler & Karkowski-Shuman, p. 545). The loss of a confidant was the only significant life event to show zero evidence of genetic covariation with major depression.

Gene-Environment Interaction.   Another study by Kendler, Kessler, et al. (1995) tested whether the risk for major depression associated with exposure to stressful life events increases significantly for those at a greater genetic risk (family history of depression) than for those with a low genetic risk (no family history). Genetic risk was indexed by assigning twin pairs to one of four categories of increasing genetic risk based on their cotwin's lifetime history: (a) MZ twin and cotwin unaffected, (b) DZ twin and cotwin unaffected, (c) DZ twin and cotwin affected, and (d) MZ twin and cotwin affected. The second set of variables was stressful life events (similar to those used in the Kendler, Neale, Kessler, Heath, & Eaves, 1993, study described previously) and a third set of variables indexed the interaction of genetic risk and stressful life events. The interaction terms consisted of a composite of the genetic risk variable and each of the stressful life events.

The genetic risk variables, stressful life events, and interaction variables were entered into a regression equation to determine the best predictors of depression. In general, Kendler, Kessler, et al. (1995) they found that interaction terms were not predictive of the onset of major depression. Rather, the best predictors of onset were: (a) any significant life event in the month that the stressful life event occurred and (b) genetic factors. Only one interaction term emerged as significant: genetic risk and "serious trouble getting along with a close relative." They concluded that, even in the presence of high genetic risk and severe stressful life events, the majority of individuals do not develop an episode of major depression and that genetic factors are important in influencing the risk of major depression in both the presence and absence of stressful life events.

The gene-environment correlation and interaction research suggests that interplay effects on depression are generally modest and that genetic and environmental effects act largely as independent main effects. However, despite identifying the genetic factors (alleles) and specific environmental factors that put individuals at high risk for depression, the onset of the disorder is by no means certain. This leaves us with the question of how these factors progress from being risk factors to precipitating illness. One mechanism of action that has been investigated is the so-called "kindling" phenomenon.

The Kindling Effect

The terms *kindling* and *kindling effect* refer to the observation that stressful life events are instrumental in the onset of major depression, but only in first-onset cases. Clinical studies have shown that the role of stressful life events decreases with recurrent depressive episodes (e.g., Brown, Harris, & Hepworth, 1994).

Kendler, Thornton, and Gardner (2000) questioned whether this is a genuine effect or a methodological artifact of the studies that report it. For example, many of the studies that reported kindling effects involved patients who were undergoing treatment for depression. As such, it is unclear if the decreasing impact of stressful life events over time is due to treatment or to patients adapting to them. Moreover, the studies are typically cross-sectional in design: First-episode patients were compared to patients who had experienced recurrent depressive episodes. This is a problem because it is unclear if the two patient groups were matched for age or sex, or even if they had experienced the same life events. What is needed is a longitudinal study where each person serves as his or her own baseline for comparison.

Accordingly, Kendler et al. (2000) conducted one to determine if the effects of significant life events genuinely diminish over time. They assessed episodes of *DSM-III-R* (1987) depression and stressful life events in a sample of 2,935 females on four separate occasions over a 9-year period. Using time-series analysis they did indeed find that the association between the stressful life events and depressive onsets diminished as the number of depressive episodes increased. In fact, they found that, for each additional depressive episode from zero to nine, the strength of association between stressful life events and depressive onsets decreased approximately 13%. As the number of previous episodes increased beyond nine, the strength of association between stressful life events and depression continued to decline but at a much slower rate (approximately 1% per episode).

Kendler et al. (2000) wrote that whatever the biological (i.e., gene transcription) or psychological processes (i.e., learning) that underlie depression are, they are "saturable." That is to say, most of the changes that occur do so in the first few episodes of the illness because the person learns to become depressed and this learning occurs intensely over the first few episodes of illness and then, with further episodes, either slows down or stops altogether (Kendler et al., 2000, pp. 1249–1250).

Do Genetic Factors Control the Kindling Effect?

What role, if any, do genetic factors play? Is the decreased effect of stressful life events on depression due to an increasing effect of genes over the environment?

Kendler et al. (2000) next tested three hypotheses about how the genetic factors might influence the kindling process: (a) genes have no effect—"the null model," (b) genes influence the speed of kindling—"the speed of kindling model," and (c) genes prime a person to be more sensitive to environmental effects—"the prekindling model." The specifics of each hypothesis are presented in Fig. 4.2.

Consistent with the prekindling model, their analyses showed that the magnitude of stressful life events and number of previous depressive episodes declined as the level of genetic risk increased. They showed this by classifying the twins into four groups of increasing genetic risk: (a) MZ twin and cotwin unaffected, (b) DZ twin and cotwin unaffected, (c) DZ twin and cotwin affected, and (d) MZ twin and cotwin affected. Individuals with no previous depressive episodes and those at highest genetic risk were shown to have a considerably weaker association between stressful life events and major depression than did those at lower genetic risk. With additional episodes, the magnitude of the association between stressful life events and the onset of major depression declined quickly in those with lowest genetic risk and hardly changed at all for those at highest risk.

Kendler et al. (2000) explained that there are distinct environmental and genetic pathways to the kindled or sensitized state in which the brain is predisposed to spontaneous depressive episodes. In the environmental pathway, an individual at low genetic risk may be exposed to a series of psychosocial adversi-

Model 1: Null model: Genes impact the overall risk for major depression; they do not influence the nature of the kindling process.

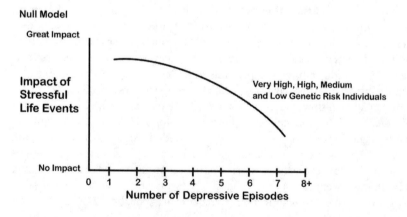

FIG. 4.2.   Three hypotheses on how genetic factors influence the environment over multiple depressive episodes. Summarized from "Stressful Life Events and Previous Episodes in the Etiology of Major Depression in Women: An Evaluation of the 'Kindling' Hypothesis," by K. Kendler, L. M. Thornton, and C. O. Gardner, 2000, *American Journal of Psychiatry, 157,* pp. 1243–1251.   *(continued on next page)*

Model 2: Speed-of-kindling model: All individuals begin with a similar degree of association between environmental adversity and risk for depressive onset, but the speed with which the kindling occurs is positively correlated with genetic risk; that is, the increasing disassociation between stressful life events and number of depressive onsets increases with genetic risk or increased heritability.

Speed-of-Kindling Model

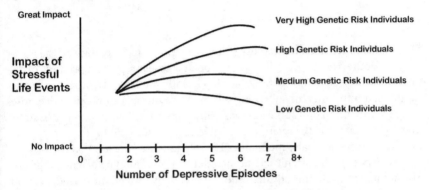

Model 3: Prekindling model: The initial strength of association between environmental adversity and risk for MDD is a function of genetic risk. Those at low genetic risk have little propensity to develop spontaneous depressive episodes and thus demonstrate a strong association between stressful life events and major depression. In contrast, those at high genetic risk would begin life prekindled, in that without previous experience with depression, they would nonetheless have a predilection to develop spontaneous depressive episodes.

Prekindling Model

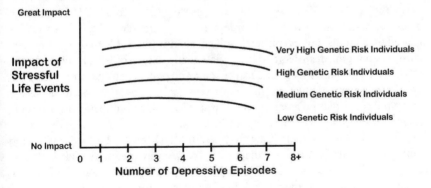

FIG. 4.2. *(continued)*

ties that precipitate a number of depressive episodes. The experience of these episodes lowers the threshold for the individual's brain to enter into the depressive state for subsequent episodes to occur with little or no environmental precipitant. Alternatively, a similar sensitized state may be reached through a genetic pathway (i.e., inheriting high risk levels) without the necessity for previous environmental exposures.

BIPOLAR DISORDER

There are relatively few heritability studies of bipolar disorder. One of the major reasons for the paucity of studies is that bipolar disorder represents a family of distinct disorders (e.g., Bipolar I, Bipolar II, Cyclothymic disorder) that are further subdivided into different subtypes, and the large number of possible diagnoses makes it difficult to find sufficient twin pairs for any statistically defensible study. The second factor is the relationship between unipolar and bipolar depression. Kendler, Pedersen, Neale, and Mathé (1995) highlighted the fact that the *DSM* diagnostic system is hierarchical: Unipolar depression cannot be diagnosed given a history of mania and thus, by definition, individuals with manic episodes are not vulnerable to unipolar depression. As a result, the unipolar and bipolar disorders are confounded and the heritability of unipolar illness cannot be sensibly estimated unless one is willing to assume that bipolar cotwins of unipolar probands (most of whom have had major depressive episodes as part of their bipolar illness) are truly affected. A similar sort of problem affects other forms of mood disorder including SAD. In the *DSM* system, SAD is a specifier to bipolar disorder or MDD, and a prerequisite to a diagnosis of SAD is preexisting unipolar or bipolar illness. This introduces a major confound into a genetic study because it will be unclear if any heritable basis or allele discovered is for bipolar depression, unipolar depression, SAD, or all three.

To circumvent this difficulty, Kendler, Pedersen, et al. (1995) estimated the heritability of *DSM-III-R* (1987) Bipolar I disorder (BP-I) and MDD as individual disorders and again as related disorders. By observing the change in heritability caused by pooling and separating the diagnoses it was possible to draw some conclusions about the disorders and their relationship to each other. The twins for this study were ascertained from Swedish hospital and population-based registries. The pooling of general population and clinical samples is noteworthy because it ensures that a full range of bipolar expression was studied while minimizing the ascertainment and sampling biases inherent in each source alone.

The study started by screening all twins for MDD and BP-I disorder. The pairs falling into either of the major diagnostic groups were then divided into narrow and broad subgroups based on their responses to a single self-report item that assessed the presence of mania and depression (yes, maybe-somewhat, no). The narrow subgroup consisted of twins that answered "yes" to having mania and depression. The broad subgroup was composed of twins that answered "yes" and "maybe-somewhat" to having experienced both mania and depression. For the broad definition of MDD and BP-I, h^2_B was estimated at 79% and 73%, respectively. The heritability of the narrow definition of MDD was 60% and 79% for BP-I. Nonshared (e^2) environmental influences made up the remainder of the variance. The finding that the heritability of BP-I and MDD was so similar suggests that they are the same disorder, with bipolar illness representing the more extreme form of affective illness.

This was tested in a follow-up analysis by estimating the heritability of combined samples of nonaffected, unipolar, and bipolar depressives. Any significant change in heritability due to the inclusion of one or more groups is suggestive of a different aetiological basis. It is important to note that this is not definitive but determines if the results are consistent with this interpretation because bipolar and unipolar depression could be influenced by different genetic factors to the same degree. The joint heritability of the narrow definition of MDD and BP-I was 64% and this increased to 83% when the broad definition was applied. When unaffected, BP-I, and MDD twin pairs were combined, the heritability of the narrow diagnostic definitions was 63%, with the estimate for the broad definition at 76%. Kendler, Pedersen, et al. (1995) concluded that the similarity of the heritability estimates across groups is consistent with the idea that bipolar and unipolar depression are influenced by a common set of genetic and environmental factors that represents a broad liability to affective illness. These findings were replicated on an American sample from Virginia (Kendler & Karkowski-Shuman, 1997), where removing bipolar pairs from a combined sample of unipolar and bipolar pairs resulted in a nonsignificant change in h^2. This study also found that mania in one twin predicts major depression in the cotwin, providing additional support for the idea that BP-I and MDD lie along a single continuum of severity and liability.

What differentiates bipolar from unipolar depression? No one is quite sure and the question has been approached by determining what is not implicated as opposed to what is. Kendler, Kessler, et al. (1995) noted that a consistent finding in twin studies of unipolar and bipolar depression is the lack of shared environmental effects (c^2), which effectively rules out hypothesized risk factors such as low social class (Brown et al., 1994; Brown, Harris, Hepworth, & Robinson, 1994), premature parental loss (Tennant, 1988), or pathogenic patterns of parental rearing (Parker, Tupling, & Brown, 1979) insofar as these affect all children in a family the same way. Current thinking in the literature suggests that it is not the action of different gene systems per se, but rather nonfamilial environmental or e^2 factors (e.g., Stancer, Persad, Wagener, & Jorna, 1987), but there is no current research that has examined specifically what kinds of environmental or experiential factors differentially influence unipolar and bipolar depression.

SEASONAL AFFECTIVE DISORDER

SAD has also been a popular phenotype for behavioral geneticists. As mentioned earlier, SAD is defined as a variant of recurrent major depression whose essential feature is the onset and remission of MDEs at characteristic times of the year

(*DSM-IV*, 1994). Typically, episodes begin in the fall or winter and remit in the spring (Rosen et al., 1990). Less commonly, there may be recurrent summer depressive episodes. Winter SAD patients usually display symptoms of depression, and several atypical symptoms such as increased appetite, overeating, and weight gain. Subclinical forms of SAD symptoms are found throughout the general population as part of everyone's normal mood variations with changes in the seasons. This is termed *seasonality*, and only the severity of response to seasonal change differentiates clinical from nonclinical samples (Blehar & Lewy, 1990). The study of seasonality greatly facilitates investigations of SAD because studies can be based on easily obtained general population study participants.

The Heritability of Seasonality and SAD

A genetic basis for SAD has been suggested by family studies of SAD patients that reported high rates of seasonal depression in first- and second-degree relatives of SAD patients (e.g., Lam, Kripke, & Gillin, 1989; Rosenthal & Wehr, 1987; White, Lewy, Sack, & Blood, 1990; Wirz-Justice, Bucheli, Schmid, & Graw, 1986). Formal heritability studies of seasonality and SAD have typically used the Seasonal Pattern Assessment Questionnaire (SPAQ). The SPAQ measures seasonal mood change in terms of the degree of seasonal variation in SAD symptoms and is widely used as a clinical screening device for SAD.

Direct evidence for genetic vulnerability was provided by Madden, Heath, Rosenthal, and Martin's (1996) analysis of 2,487 general population Australian twin pairs who completed the SPAQ. Multivariate genetic analyses showed that a single set of genetic influences exerted a global influence across seasonal changes in eating, sleeping, weight change, socializing, energy level, and mood. At the level of individual symptoms, the strongest genetic influences were found for items measuring changes in mood and energy levels. These items are summarized in the Global Seasonality Score, whose heritability was estimated at a modest 29% in both males and females.

Madden et al.'s (1996) results raise two questions. First, although the heritability of seasonality in males and females was estimated at 29%, this does not automatically mean that the same genetic and environmental factors are operating in both genders because there are marked gender differences in severity and prevalence (e.g., Rosen et al., 1990). Second, the results of the Australian twin study may not be generalizable to populations in the northern hemisphere, such as Canada. Some studies suggest that the severity of SAD and seasonality varies with latitude and possibly climate (e.g., Okawa et al., 1996) but others have reported that the symptoms of SAD in different hemispheres are similar (e.g., Boyce & Parker, 1988) and that seasonal sensitivity is not affected by latitude (e.g., Muscettola et al., 1995).

Jang, Lam, Livesley, and Vernon (1997) administered the SPAQ to 339 twin pairs from British Columbia, Canada. In contrast to the Australian study, the heritability of the Global Seasonality Score was 69% in males and 45% in females. Similar to the Australian samples, individual symptoms, including changes in sleep patterns, social activities, mood, appetite, and energy levels, primarily had the highest heritability in both males (median = 45.5%) and females (median = 30.5%). For both sexes, weight changes were not heritable and sex-by-genotype analyses suggested that the genetic factors that influence female seasonality are not the same as those that influenced male seasonality but that the environmental influences (specifically the e^2 influences) were common to both genders.

One explanation for the differences between the Canadian and Australian samples is that the Australian study may have underestimated heritability, because of the lower prevalence rates of the disorder or reduced range in the severity of reported symptoms due to the milder climate in Australia. The Australian sample reported fewer seasonal problems than the Canadian sample (13% vs. 33.6%), and lower rates of SAD as indicated by the SPAQ criteria (2% vs. 9.8%).

The differences in prevalence and severity of seasonality and SAD in males and females, coupled with the differences in heritability, provide some insight into what the purpose of seasonality or SAD genes might be. Genetic studies typically assume that genetic factors increase the risk or vulnerability to disorder. The lower prevalence and severity of seasonality among males from the general population (e.g., Rosen et al., 1990) suggests, however, that specific genetic factors in males may increase their resistance to the impact of seasonal change. The evolution of such a protective mechanism in males would have conferred an adaptive advantage to those who possessed the appropriate resistance genes.

Early human societies were small hunter-gatherer units with a clear division of labor between females and males (e.g., Trivers, 1985). The male contribution to the family resources would be to provide foodstuffs through hunting, which must occur throughout all seasons. The role of females involved the gathering of foodstuffs and agriculture, activities that are tied to the seasons. As such, a clear fitness advantage in males was conferred if they were not affected by seasonal changes, whereas females' fitness was enhanced if their activities were influenced by changes in the seasons. The ancestral environments in which these adaptations have evolved no longer exist, rendering them obsolete, but evolution is a long process and these once-useful adaptations have become liabilities in our modern world.

SUMMARY

At present, linkage and association studies have yet to produce replicable findings that would have immediate benefits for clinical practice. Heritability analyses have shown the depressive phenotype to be differentially heritable. The heritability of severe depression typical of clinically depressed patients has been found to be 70% or more. The heritability of less severe forms of depression typical of general population samples falls within the 30% to 40% range. When the analysis is applied to individual depressive symptoms, some symptoms such as feelings of loneliness, crying, interpersonal problems, nausea, and headaches, which represent reactions to stressful life events or changes in body function, appear to be even less heritable compared to endogenous symptoms (e.g., sleep disturbances, libido, appetite, loss of energy, and personality). Moreover, the etiological pathways to depression appear to be gender-specific.

Behavioral genetic studies of BP-I disorder suggest that bipolar illness is a highly heritable (60%– 70%) extreme form of unipolar illness. The evidence supports the hypothesis that the disorders occupy different points along a single continuum of liability for a broader concept of affective illness. The continuity between the two disorders is likely due to the action of the same genetic factors, but what differentiates bipolar from unipolar illness is the operation of environmental influences specific to each form but these remain to be identified. Other forms of depression such as SAD have also been shown to have a significant heritable basis that may vary by latitude or prevalence of the disorder. Greater genetic variation is observed in populations from northern as opposed to southern latitudes.

Genetic and environmental effects appear to operate largely as main effects. To date, little evidence for gene-environment interplay has been reported. The primary predictors of the onset of major depression are: stressful life events in the past year, genetic factors, previous history of major depression, and the personality trait of neuroticism. The role of genetic factors has been shown to sensitize some people to the influence of depressogenic events, in particular, stressful live events that lead to first-episode depression. The role of stressful life events has been shown to slowly diminish over time as people learn to be depressed, or habituate to a depressed state. This suggests that it is possible to teach patients to break the depressive cycle as a key element in their treatment.

Chapter 5

The Personality Disorders

There is little disagreement among personality disorder researchers that normal and abnormal personality are related but there is little agreement as to why they are related.

—Widiger, Verheul, and van den Brink (1999)

Some of the earliest behavioral genetic research focused on personality constructs. Over this long history, an extensive body of research has covered the heritability of personality traits and has started to address some of the central issues in this field, including: (a) the validity of the dimensional model of personality and its disorders, (b) the definition of the major personality domains, and (c) the number of personality disorder diagnoses. This chapter illustrates how behavioral genetic research has been used to address these issues.

THE DIMENSIONAL MODEL OF PERSONALITY

Types or Traits?

A central problem of personality disorder research is the validity of the dimensional model of personality disorder, which states that personality disorder represents the extremes of normal personality function. Individual differences in personality function are not a reflection of which traits an individual may or may not possess, but rather on which traits a person scores most highly. That is to say, all individuals possess a universal set of traits and are distinguished by the salience of particular traits; disorder is defined by the trait(s) whose expression exceeds an accepted population norm.

The dimensional model does not allow for the existence of personality types such as the "Type A and B personalities" or the "addictive personality," which have been posited throughout the history of psychology and psychiatry. In so doing, the dimensional model challenges the validity of the personality disorder diagnoses contained in the *DSM-IV* (1994) Axis II, whose labels divide personality into quasitypes such as "borderline" or "schizoid." A compelling reason for the growing interest in dimensional models is that diagnostic types such as these seldom adequately capture the complete clinical presentation. Often the presenting patient fails to meet a few diagnostic criteria or exhibits behavior that falls outside the circumscribed limits of a type.

The very fact that the *DSM-IV* (1994) permits the assignment of multiple diagnoses to ensure that all aspects of a patient's clinical presentation are captured implicitly suggests that personality function is best described and measured with a trait-based approach! Despite the appeal of the dimensional model, there remain several questions to be resolved before it can have an impact on the way in which personality disorder is assessed and diagnosed. They are: (a) How many traits? (b) How are they organized? and (c) what causes scores in the normal range to move to the extreme range?

Models of Personality

According to the dimensional model, personality disorder represents the extremes of normal personality function. Thus, the best place to start to answer the previous questions is with the behavioral genetic analysis of normal personality. In the past decade, personality researchers have reached the conclusion that virtually all measures of personality can be reduced to five basic personality domains: neuroticism (N), extraversion (E), openness to experience (O), agreeableness (A), and conscientiousness (C). This is called the "Five-Factor Model of Personality" (FFM: Passini & Norman, 1966) or the "Big Five." Neuroticism refers to chronic levels of emotional adjustment. Extraversion refers to the quantity and intensity of preferred interpersonal interactions, activity level, need for adjustment, stimulation, and capacity for joy. Openness to experience describes the active seeking and appreciation of experiences for their own sake. Agreeableness is an interpersonal dimension that refers to types of preferred interactions along a continuum of compassion to antagonism. Conscientiousness refers to a person's degree of organization, persistence, control, and motivation and goal-directed behavior (Costa & Widiger, 1994). A great deal of phenotypic research shows how other models of personality such as Eysenck and Eysenck's (1992) psychoticism (P), extraversion (E), and neuroticism (N) model (or the PEN model, also called the "Gigantic Three") and the FFM are related in predictable ways. For example, their conceptions of neuroticism and extraversion are highly similar, and psychoticism has a well-established and predictable negative relationship to agreeableness (Larstone, Jang, Livesley, Vernon, & Wolf, 2002).

The Heritability of Normal and Abnormal Personality Function

Heritability analyses of the five domains have produced one of the most replicated results in psychology: Between 40% and 50% of the total variability on each trait is attributable to additive genetic factors (h^2_A), little or none is due to shared (c^2) environmental factors, and the remainder is accounted for by nonshared (e^2) environmental factors (e.g., Bouchard & Loehlin, 2001).

Heritability studies of personality disorder traits have yielded similar results. Personality disorder trait scales differ from measures of normal personality in that their item content assesses more extreme forms of behavior. A classic measure of this type is the Minnesota Multiphasic Personality Inventory (MMPI: Greene, 1991). DiLalla, Carey, Gottesman, and Bouchard (1996) estimated the heritability of the ten standard MMPI clinical scales on a sample of 65 MZ and 54 DZ twin pairs who were separated as infants and raised apart. The heritability (h^2_B) estimates were: hypochondriasis (35%), depression (31%), hysteria (26%), psychopathic deviate (61%), masculinity-femininity (36%), paranoia (28%), psychasthenia (60%), schizophrenia (61%), hypomania (55%), and social introversion (34%).

The original MMPI items have been the subject of controversy with respect to their validity and reliability. A major revision of the items known as "Wiggins' Content Scales" (see Greene, 1991; and Wiggins, 1966; for a description) is significant because the new scales have demonstrated content validity, no item overlap, and they cover a wide range of thoughts, experiences, and behaviors associated with psychopathology. DiLalla and colleagues estimated the heritability of these scales at: social maladjustment (27%), depression (44%), feminine interests (36%), poor morale (39%), religious fundamentalism (57%), authority conflict (42%), psychoticism (62%), organic symptoms (42%), family problems (50%), manifest hostility (37%), phobias (59%), hypomania (45%), and poor health (56%). Over these two sets of scales, the median heritability was 44%, which falls within the same range as normal personality.

Another measure that has been subjected to extensive heritability analysis is the Dimensional Assessment of Personality Pathology (DAPP: Livesley & Jackson, in press). The traits for this scale were developed from an extensive review of the personality disorder literature and identified by panels of clinicians who were asked to identify the most prototypical features of each *DSM-III-R* (1987) personality disorder diagnosis (Livesley, 1985a, 1985b; 1986; Livesley, Jackson, & Schroeder, 1989). This work yielded eighteen traits that have been validated across samples of personality-disordered patients and the general population. Consistent with the dimensional model, the same eighteen traits are found in both clinical and general population samples. The only difference is that patients score higher on the traits than nonpatients.

The heritability (h^2_A) of the eighteen DAPP scales in a general population sample was estimated at: affective lability (45%), anxiousness (44%), callousness (56%), cognitive distortion (49%), compulsivity (37%), conduct problems (56%), identity problems (53%), insecure attachment (48%), intimacy problems (48%), narcissism (53%), oppositionality (46%), rejection (35%), restricted expression (50%), self-harm (41%), social avoidance (53%), stimulus seeking (40%), submissiveness (45%), and suspiciousness (45%) (Jang, Livesley, Vernon, & Jackson, 1996). Like the MMPI, the estimates of heritability for the DAPP are congruent with those obtained with measures of normal personality function.

The eighteen DAPP traits can be reduced to four higher order factors (e.g., Larstone et al., 2002). The first factor, emotional dysregulation, represents unstable and reactive tendencies, dissatisfaction with the self and life experiences, and interpersonal problems. This factor subsumes the personality trait of neuroticism and reflects the essential features of *DSM-IV* (1994) borderline personality disorder. The second factor is dissocial behavior because it resembles antisocial personality disorder and is negatively related to agreeableness. The third factor is inhibition. This factor is negatively related to extraversion and resembles avoidant and schizoid personality disorders. The fourth factor, compulsivity, is positively related to the trait of conscientiousness and clearly resembles obsessive-compulsive personality disorder. These four factors are important because they establish a predictable link between the domains of normal and abnormal personality functioning.

Heritability analysis (h^2_A) of emotional dysregulation was 52%, dissocial was 50%, inhibition 50% and compulsivity was 44% with nonshared effects accounting for the remainder (Jang, Livesley, & Vernon, 1996). The phenotypic correspondence between the primary domains of abnormal and normal personality and similarity of heritability estimates provide strong circumstantial support for the validity of the dimensional model.

Four Unsolved Puzzles in the Heritability of Personality Function

Despite the consistency of heritability estimates across different personality scales, there remain four puzzles. The first is that the heritability of clinically diagnosed personality disorder is not really known. Unlike other psychopathologies, heritability studies of twin pairs with diagnosed personality disorders are virtually nonexistent. The second puzzle is the fleeting influence of nonadditive genetic effects (h^2_d). Some studies find evidence of genetic nonadditivity whereas others do not. The third puzzle is gender. Some studies have shown that the heritability of personality traits in females is greater than in males, but the finding has not been consistently replicated. It is unclear if these puzzles are the result of methodological problems or if they reflect important aetiological differences in personality.[1]

Puzzle 1: The Heritability of Diagnosed Personality Disorder.   The few detailed reviews of the genetics of personality disorder (e.g., Dahl, 1993; McGuffin & Thapar, 1992; Nigg & Goldsmith, 1994; Thapar & McGuffin, 1993) concluded that personality disorder is heritable. Unfortunately, these conclusions are largely ex-

---

[1]The fourth is there an etiological basis underlying the relationship between normal and abnormal personality.

trapolations from heritability studies of clinical scales applied to healthy twins. Heritability studies of diagnosed personality disorder are rare, and the few that exist are based on small samples (e.g., fewer than twenty pairs) or on patients who present with comorbid conditions that confound results.

For example, Torgersen, Lygren, and Oien (2000) found that heritability of borderline personality disorder was 69%. However, the sample was extremely small and consisted of 17 monozygotic and 31 dizygotic pairs. An earlier study by Torgersen, Skre, Onstad, Edvardsen, and Kringlen (1993) estimated the heritability of *DSM-III-R* (1987) personality disorder criteria using healthy twin pairs whose relatives were also diagnosed with schizophrenia. Personality disorder criteria were assessed and ratings were subjected to factor analysis. Twelve factors were extracted. Heritability (h^2_B) was: self-effacive (63%), affect-constricted (38%), contrary (30%), perfectionistic (30%), suspicious (27%), egocentric (24%), appealing (12%), disorganized (2%), insecure (4%), seclusive (0%), unreliable (4%), and submissive (0%). It is unclear if the results are tapping into the liability for schizophrenia or some other disorder that the family members share. In contrast, family studies of personality disorder suggest that the diagnoses are highly familial. In a recent family study of borderline personality disorder (BPD), White, Gunderson, and Zanarini (2003) estimated the prevalence of BPD in relatives of probands is four to twenty times higher than the estimated rate in the general population. However, this rate can vary dramatically depending on whether the diagnosis was made by directly interviewing each family member.

Given the difficulty finding twins that meet the diagnostic criteria for personality disorder, a growing trend in research is to conduct heritability studies of specific traits associated with personality dysfunction. Recent examples include twin studies of aggression (Seroczynski, Bergeman, & Coccaro, 1999; Vernon, McCarthy, Johnson, Jang, & Harris, 1999), "pre-schizophrenic personality" (van Kampen, 1999), and juvenile antisocial traits (Lyons, True, Eisen, & Goldberg, 1995). However, many of these scales were developed by the laboratory that conducted the study. As such, they have not been subjected to widespread use and thus, relatively little is known about their reliability and validity.

Puzzle 2: Genetic Nonadditivity. The second puzzle is the fleeting influence of nonadditive genetic effects (h^2_d). Bouchard (1997) reported that nonadditive effects were not present in the research reports generated by the Minnesota study of twins reared apart. In contrast, studies of twins reared together (e.g., Loehlin, 1986, 1992; Loehlin, Horn, & Willermann, 1997; Loehlin & Nichols, 1976) reported that these effects accounted for a sizeable portion of the total genetic contribution. This suggests that differences in study methodology may be the cause.

Nonadditive results also seem to appear as a function of the personality measure. For example, Waller and Shaver (1994) and Finkel and McGue (1997) reported finding nonadditive genetic effects on the Multidimensional Personality Questionnaire (MPQ: Tellegen, 1982) scales administered to samples of twins reared together. However, nonadditive effects have rarely, if ever, been reported on direct measures of the FFM such as Costa & McCrae's (1992) Revised Neuroticism Extraversion Openness Personality Inventory (NEO-PI-R) used in studies of twins reared together (e.g., Jang et al., 1996; Jang, McCrae, Angleitner, Riemann, & Livesley, 1998; Riemann, Angleitner, & Strelau, 1997).

Puzzle 3: Gender. The third puzzle is gender. Rose (1988) reported greater female heritability on the MMPI scales for psychoticism, masculinity, somatic complaints, and intellectual differences. Zonderman (1982) found the same for the responsibility, achievement via independence, and femininity scales of the California Personality Inventory (CPI: Gough, 1989). Finkel and McGue (1997) also reported higher female heritability for the MPQ absorption scale, but male heritability was higher for the alienation and control scales.

Eaves, Eysenck, and Martin (1989) reported that the heritability of EPQ neuroticism and extraversion was higher in females than males. However, Loehlin's (1992) combined analysis of the twin data obtained from major studies of personality suggested that the heritability of neuroticism and extraversion was higher among males. Macaskill, Hopper, White, and Hill (1994) did not find significant sex differences in neuroticism but did find the heritability of extraversion to be significantly higher among males. It is quite possible that differential heritability according to gender is due to the fact that different genes influence personality in males and females; sex-limitation analyses can help resolve this issue.

Finkel and McGue (1997) simultaneously analyzed personality data obtained on twins and their parents and siblings. Their extensive set of analyses showed that genetic influences that underlie female MPQ traits also influence male scores on eleven of the fourteen scales. The exceptions were alienation, control, and absorption, for which different gender-specific genetic influences were detected. For all fourteen scales they found that the same environmental factors (e^2) influence both genders to varying degrees.

Unfortunately, some of these findings are undermined by inconsistencies in the twin correlations. For example, the correlation for DZ male, female, and opposite-sex pairs for social potency are 0.33, 0.28, and 0.16, respectively. Note that the correlation for the opposite-sex pairs is about half the size of either same-sex correlation. Significant differences in the opposite-sex pair correlations compared to the same-sex pairs is an indication that sex-specific effects are present. Another inconsistency is that, although sex-specific effects were reported for absorption, the magnitudes of the same and opposite-sex pair twin correlations did not differ (e.g., $r_{\text{DZ Males}} = 0.17$, $r_{\text{DZ Females}} = 0.13$, and $r_{\text{DZ Opposite-sex}} = 0.16$). A possible explanation for the inconsistencies between the twin correlations and the model-fitting analyses is that their analyses were not based solely on twin data but also incorporated data from their families.

In a study that used only twin data, Jang, Livesley, and Vernon (1998) applied sex-limitation analyses to the eighteen DAPP scales. The sample consisted of 681 volunteer general population twin pairs (128 monozygotic male, 208 monozygotic female, 75 dizygotic male, 174 dizygotic female, 96 dizygotic opposite-sex pairs).

The first set of analyses estimated the heritability of the scales in males and females separately. Among females, all DAPP scales except cognitive distortion, compulsivity, conduct problems, suspiciousness, and self-harm were heritable. Among males only submissiveness did not have a significant heritability. Sex-limitation analyses showed that the genes influencing stimulus seeking, callousness, rejection, and insecure attachment were common to males and females. The genetic factors influencing the remaining fourteen scales were clearly unique to each gender. However, like Finkel and McGue (1997), the environmental factors (e^2) that influenced one gender also influenced the other.

In general, the Finkel and McGue (1997) study of normal personality traits found far less evidence of gender-specific genetic factors than the Jang, Livesley, and Vernon (1998) study of personality disorder traits. Taken at face value, this finding suggests that gender differences in the prevalence of personality disorder (known to be greater in females) may be due to the action of gender-specific genetic factors. The alternative explanation is that the difference between the two studies is no more than a methodological artifact. For example, it could be argued that the MPQ is not sensitive enough to detect sex differences because its scales assess both positive and negative aspects of personality. The DAPP is more specific because it focuses solely on the pathological aspects of personality function. This specificity may have provided the sensitivity necessary to detect sex differences, a potentially important factor noted by Loehlin (1982).

Puzzle 4: The Relationship Between Normal and Abnormal Personality. In the opening sentence of this chapter, I noted that there is agreement that normal and abnormal personality are related, but little agreement as to why. Some direct evidence that the two domains share a common genetic basis has been provided by multivariate genetic studies. For example, Jang and Livesley (1999) estimated the genetic correlations between the short version of the NEO-PI-R (Costa & McCrae, 1992) and the eighteen DAPP scales using data from a sample of 545 volunteer general population twin pairs. Several large genetic correlations were found between NEO neuroticism and DAPP anxiousness ($r_G = .81$), submissiveness ($r_G = .61$), cognitive distortion ($r_G = .76$), identity problems ($r_G = .78$), and affective lability ($r_G = .73$) scales. DAPP social avoidance ($r_G = -.65$) was found to share a common genetic basis with NEO extraversion, whereas DAPP callousness ($r_G = -.65$), suspiciousness ($r_G = -.57$), and rejection sensitivity ($r_G = -.54$) were found to share a common genetic basis with NEO agreeableness. DAPP conscientiousness ($r_G = .52$) and passive-oppositional behavior ($r_G = -.76$) were found to be in a pleiotropic relationship with NEO conscientiousness. In contrast, virtually all of the genetic correlations between the DAPP dimensions and NEO openness to experience were small, ranging from −.17 to .20 (median $r_G = -.04$), which is not surprising given that these types of behaviors are not observed in personality disordered populations. In contrast to the genetic correlations between the DAPP and NEO-PI-R scales, the environmental correlations were uniformly low and were much more specific to each domain.

Markon, Krueger, Bouchard, and Gottesman (2002) found the same pattern of relationships between the MMPI and MPQ completed by 128 MZ pairs of twins reared apart. Their first analysis estimated the genetic correlations between the lower order MMPI and MPQ scales. Substantial genetic correlations were found between MPQ stress, alienation, and absorption scales and nearly all of the MMPI scales (r_G range = .47 to .96). Their second analysis separately factored the MMPI and MPQ scales to extract higher order scores for each instrument and estimated genetic correlations between them. The genetic correlations between the MPQ positive emotionality, negative emotionality, and constraint and MMPI ego control were –.40, –.18 (ns), and .57, respectively. The genetic correlation between the MMPI ego resiliency and the MPQ positive emotionality, negative emotionality, and constraint was –.11 (ns), –.86, and –.09 (ns), respectively. The environmental correlations between the MPQ and MMPI higher order dimensions were uniformly low.

Has a Dimensional Model of Personality Disorder Been Supported?   The behavioral genetic literature has certainly produced evidence consistent with predictions made by the dimensional model. The strongest evidence is that the heritability estimates for measures of normal and abnormal personality are very similar, suggesting that they share a common genetic aetiology. This common aetiology has been verified by multivariate genetic research between measures of normal and abnormal personality. The major limitation of this research is that the assessment of personality disorder used in these studies has relied on measures that assess extreme personality function and that have been administered to general population subjects.

THE DEFINITION OF THE MAJOR PERSONALITY DOMAINS

From the preceding section, it should be clear that many different models of personality exist as evidenced by the large number of different scales employed. I highlighted work on the MPQ, EPQ-R, NEO-PI-R, DAPP, MMPI, and others. Why do personality researchers keep inventing different scales? In the beginning of this chapter I mentioned that all of these measures encompass some or all of the Big Five personality dimensions. Despite general agreement on what N, E, A, O, and C are, there remain questions about the specifics.

For example, Depue and Collins (1999) reviewed the definition of extraversion as assessed by the major scales. They found that all of the scales recognized sociability and affiliation, but not all recognized agency (e.g., surgency, exhibitionism), activation (e.g., activity level), impulsivity or sensation seeking (e.g., novelty seeking, monotony avoidance), positive emotions (e.g., enthusiasm, cheerfulness), or optimism. Similarly, the NEO-PI-R neuroticism scale (Costa & McCrae, 1992) contains items assessing impulsive behaviors, but these are not measured by the EPQ-R neuroticism construct (Eysenck & Eysenck, 1992), indicating that the definition of the neuroticism trait is fundamentally different in each model. This issue is the problem of domain content.

Related to this issue is the problem of how these domains are organized, or the problem of trait structure. Presently, it is assumed that the subtraits defining a domain are organized in terms of a strict hierarchy in which each domain is composed of a specific set of subtraits (e.g., NEO-PI-R conscientiousness is composed of six subtraits or *facets*: competence, order, dutifulness, achievement striving, self-discipline, and deliberation). Domains are also assumed to be additive in nature—scores on each of the subtraits can be summed to yield a measure of the domain.

This hierarchy suggests that each subtrait defining a domain must derive a significant proportion of its genetic influence from the larger domain and that the search for putative genes should be directed at the level of the domain. As a result, by finding the genes for a domain one will have found the genes for each of the subtraits defining the domain. A clinical implication of this hierarchy is that focusing treatment on one subtrait will automatically impact all the others. Similarly, if one subtrait is difficult to modify, then it can be influenced to some degree by focusing attention on a more accessible subtrait. A central question of personality research is whether personality traits are organized in this hierarchical structure.

Multivariate genetic models such as the independent and common pathways models simultaneously address the problems of domain content and structure. For example, NEO-PI-R neuroticism as defined by its six facets is shown in Fig. 5.1 (a). An alternative organization is shown in Fig. 5.1 (b). These figures are instantly recognizable as the common and independent pathways models and the relative fit of each to the data addresses questions on domain structure. Questions of domain content are addressed by the degree to which the subtraits share a common genetic basis. A case could be made, for example, that impulsivity is not a facet of neuroticism by demonstrating that only a small proportion of its genetic influence is common to the remaining five subtraits.

Jang, Livesley, Angleitner, Riemann, and Vernon (2002) used common and independent pathways models to study the structure and content of the five NEO-PI-R domains. The models were applied separately to a sample of 253 identical and 207 fraternal twin pairs from Canada and 526 identical and 269 fraternal pairs from Germany, providing a test of the generalizability of the genetic and environmental structure across cultures. For each sample, a single-factor common pathways model (as illustrated in Fig. 5.1 [a]) and a series of independent pathways models (Fig. 5.1 [b]) was tested. Shared environmental effects (c^2) were omitted from all models because previous heritability analyses of the personality trait scales showed that these effects were minimal. The model-fitting analyses rejected the common pathways model for all domains.

Instead, an independent pathways model specifying two additive genetic factors and two nonshared environmental factors provided the best fit in both samples. Representative results are presented in Fig. 5.2 and Fig. 5.3. The failure of the common pathways model is significant because it suggests that, despite the fact that all facets share a common genetic basis to some degree, the symmetrical hierarchical structure avidly sought by trait theorists and students of psychopathology does not exist.

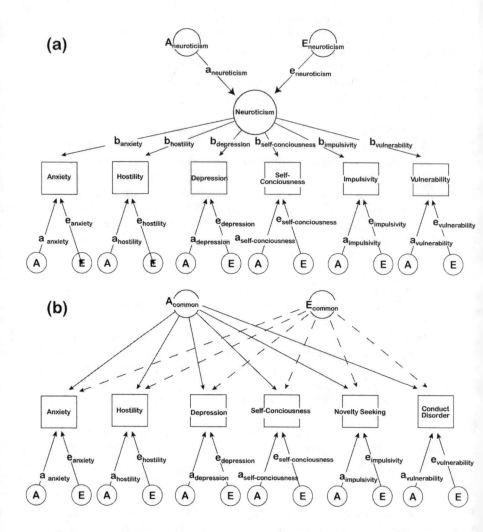

FIG. 5.1.   Hypothetical organization of neuroticism.

Johnson and Krueger (in press) reported similar results with a set of adjectives used to describe personality (e.g., outgoing, lively, nervous, etc.) that were subjected to multivariate genetic modeling. They asked 315 monozygotic and 275 same-sex dizygotic twin pairs from the National Survey of Midlife Development in the United States to rate themselves on each of the adjectives. For the adjectives describing neuroticism and extraversion, a common pathways model provided a good fit. In contrast, for the adjectives describing agreeableness, conscientiousness, and openness the independent pathways model provided the best fit.

Implications for Trait Structure

The fact that the common pathways model does not consistently provide a good explanation for the structure of major personality domains suggests that there are no genes for N, E, O, A, and C per se. Rather, higher order traits are simply a convenient heuristic to describe the action of genes consistent with the lexical view of Saucier and Goldberg (1996), who argued that the five domains are merely a convenient way of organizing lower order traits. Moreover, the finding that more than one genetic factor is required to account for the relationship between subtraits, as per the independent pathways model, supports the idea that there is no inherent reason to assume that domains are equal in breadth or pervasiveness.

A third finding is that the subtraits of a domain have a distinct heritable component unique to each, indicating that they are not merely facets of broader traits but rather distinct heritable entities themselves. In fact, once Jang, McCrae, Angleitner, Riemann, and Livesley (1998) corrected the NEO-PI-R scales for unreliability (raw heritability estimate divided by the test-retest reliability), the residual heritability (h^2_A) on the thirty subtraits became quite substantial and ranged from 25% (competence) to 65% (dutifulness). Livesley, Jang, and Vernon (1998) reported similar findings for measures of personality disorder. The heritability unique to each of the eighteen DAPP subscales ranged from .26 (intimacy problems) to .48 (conduct problems). Findings such as these raise the possibility that not all traits are organized into clusters of covarying features but retain relatively distinct characteristics.

Implications for Domain Content

The magnitude of the parameter estimates show that the proportion of the genetic influences shared by all subtraits is quite variable. For example, in Fig. 5.2, the subtrait of impulsivity was the least influenced by common genetic factors compared to other subtraits. In the Canadian twin sample, 34% of this subtrait's variability was attributable to the first genetic factor. In the German twin sample, only 15% was accounted for by the first genetic factor. In both samples, most of the variability of this subtrait was directly due to the action of genes unique to impulsivity (66% in the Canadian sample and 88% in the German sample). This kind of information can be used to argue that impulsivity should not be considered an aspect of neuroticism.

Indeed, it can be argued that impulsivity has more in common with extraversion. This is an empirical question that could be determined by jointly analyzing all six extraversion facets with impulsivity. The best test would be to subject all twelve extraversion and neuroticism facets to joint analysis to determine which subtraits share a common aetiology. This is a study that has yet to be done with the NEO-PI-R. A good example of the utility of this strategy, however, was presented by Ando et al. (2004) who applied it to Cloninger's Temperament and Character Inventory (TCI).

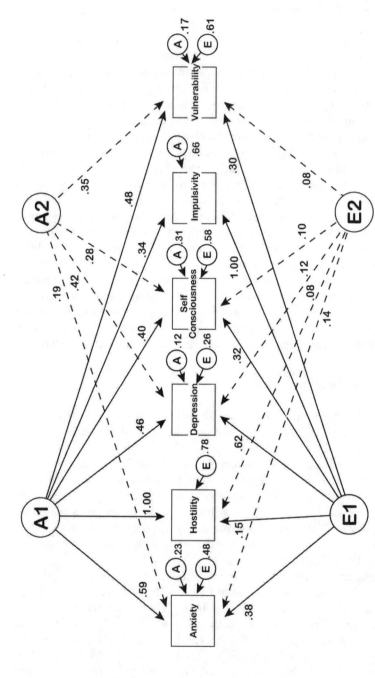

FIG. 5.2a.   Multivariate genetic structure of NEO-PI-R neuroticism in a sample of Canadian twins.

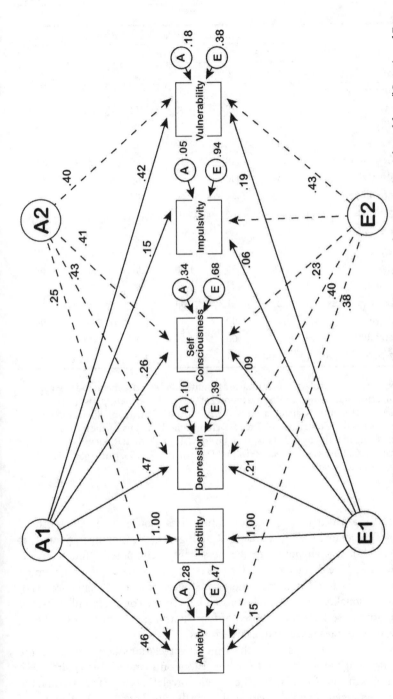

FIG. 5.2b. Multivariate genetic structure of NEO-PI-R neuroticism in a sample of Canadian and German twins. Adapted from "Genetic and Environmental Influences on the Covariance of Facets Defining the Domains of the Five-Factor Model of Personality," by K. L. Jang, W. J. Livesley, A. Angleither, R. Riemann, and P. A. Vernon, 2002, *Personality and Individual Differences, 33*, p. 94. Copyright 2002 by Elsevier Science. Adapted with permission.

NYACK COLLEGE MANHATTAN

99

Facet Scale	Variance Accounted by Each Parameter					
	A		E			
	1	2	1	2	A′	E′
Canadian Sample						
Anxiety	.59	.19	.38	.14	.23	.48
Hostility	1.00	.00	.15	.08	.00	.78
Depression	.46	.42	.62	.12	.12	.26
Self-Consciousness	.40	.28	.32	.10	.31	.58
Impulsivity	.34	.00	1.00	.00	.66	.00
Vulnerability	.48	.35	.30	.08	.17	.61

$\chi^2 = 152.30$, $p = .05$, $df = 125$, RMSEA = .025, 90% UL = .042, AIC = −97.70

German Sample						
Anxiety	.45	.25	.15	.38	.28	.47
Hostility	1.00	.00	1.00	.00	.00	.00
Depression	.47	.43	.21	.40	.10	.39
Self-Consciousness	.26	.41	.09	.23	.34	.68
Impulsivity	.15	.00	.06	.00	.85	.94
Vulnerability	.42	.00	.19	.43	.18	.38

$\chi^2 = 137.76$, $p = .22$, $df = 126$, RMSEA = .011, 90% UL = .027, AIC = −114.24

FIG. 5.3. Proportions of the total variance accounted for by each genetic and environmental factor (independent pathways model) of the NEO-PI-R neuroticism facets on samples of German and Canadian twins. Adapted from "Genetic and Environmental Influences on the Covariance of Facets Defining the Domains of the Five-Factor Model of Personality," by K. L. Jang, W. J. Livesley, A. Angleitner, R. Riemann, and P. A. Vernon, 2002, *Personality and Individual Differences, 33*, p. 94. Copyright 2002 by Elsevier Science. Adapted with permission.

The TCI is a 240-item scale that operationalizes Cloninger's Psychobiosocial Model of Temperament and Character (Cloninger, 1986; Cloninger, Svrakic, & Przybeck, 1993), which hypothesizes that personality is composed of four temperament traits and three character traits. Of interest here are three of the temperament traits: novelty seeking (NS), harm avoidance (HA), and reward dependence (RD). Like most personality scales, each dimension is composed of several subtraits. For example, novelty seeking is composed of four subtraits: exploratory excitability, impulsiveness, extravagance, and disorderliness.

Ando et al. (2004) computed the genetic correlations between all of the subtraits defining the NS, HA, and RD dimensions on a sample of 414 pairs of MZ and 203 DZ twin pairs from Japan. The genetic correlations were factored and the factors that emerged did not quite resemble the designed phenotypic structure of NS, HA, and RD (see Fig. 5.4). The first genetic factor suggested that the subtrait

	I	II	III	IV
Novelty seeking				
Exploratory excitability	**.62**	.28	.25	.29
Impulsiveness	-.10	.03	.03	**.76**
Extravagance	.02	.16	.00	**.72**
Disorderliness	.03	-.16	.15	**.74**
Harm Avoidance				
Anticipatory worry	**-.87**	.01	-.03	-.01
Fear of uncertainty	**-.51**	.28	-.32	**-.43**
Shyness	**-.76**	-.16	-.22	-.05
Fatigability	**-.72**	-.26	-.06	-.10
Reward dependence				
Sentimentality	-.06	**.56**	**.60**	-.04
Attachment	.04	**.70**	.00	.22
Dependence	-.09	**.86**	-.19	.13

FIG. 5.4. Varimax rotated principal factor analysis loading matrix of the genetic correlations estimated between the TCI temperament subscales. Adapted from "Genetic and Environmental Structure of Cloninger's Temperament and Character Dimensions," by J. Ando et al., 2004, *Journal of Personality Disorders, 18*, p. 387. Copyright 2004 by Guilford Publications. Adapted with permission.

of exploratory excitability shared more genes with harm avoidance. Factor II resembled Cloninger's reward dependence as originally designed. Factor III suggested that novelty seeking should only include the facets of impulsiveness, extravagance, and disorderliness.

Using this information, the Harm Avoidance scale (*r*-HA) was revised to consist of exploratory excitability, anticipatory worry, fear of uncertainty, shyness, and fatigability. Novelty seeking (*r*-NS) was revised to consist of impulsiveness, extravagance, and disorderliness. RD was left intact. The genetic and environmental correlations computed between *r*-NS, *r*-HA, and RD were very small (ranging from –.02 to .11), indicating that the revised temperament scales are now genetically homogeneous and independent. Findings such as these demonstrate the utility of behavioral genetic analyses to address central questions of how personality is structured and how its traits are defined.

THE NUMBER OF PERSONALITY TRAITS AND DIAGNOSES

It is odd that personality research consistently finds five broad domains of personality, yet there are currently ten personality disorder diagnoses. The fact that normal and abnormal personality disorders have been shown to share a common genetic aetiology suggests that only five diagnoses may be valid. Or, could the actual number of diagnoses be about three? The *DSM* suggests this by organizing the ten diagnoses into three clusters (akin to personality domains) because they share common phenotypic features. The three clusters are: Cluster A (paranoid, schizoid, schizotypal personality disorder diagnoses), representing odd and eccentric features; Cluster B (antisocial, borderline, histrionic, narcissistic personality disorder diagnoses), representing dramatic, emotional, and erratic features; and Cluster C (avoidant, dependent, and obsessive-compulsive personality disorder diagnoses), representing anxious and fearful features. It is interesting to note that each of these three clusters reflect to some extent at least one of the five major personality domains. However, there is little one-to-one correspondence between the Big Five and the clusters. Cluster B, for example, resembles a combination of features from neuroticism, extraversion (−), and agreeableness (−) from the Big Five.

Behavioral geneticists have attempted to address this issue by estimating the genetic and environmental correlations between all subtraits of a measure and subjecting them to factor analysis to determine why subscales sort themselves into broad domains. For example, in two independent samples of twins, McCrae, Jang, Livesley, Riemann, and Angleitner (2001) estimated the genetic and environmental correlations between all 30 of the NEO-PI-R facets on twins recruited in Germany and Canada. Factor analysis of these r_G and r_E matrices yielded five factors that were clearly recognizable as N, E, O, A, and C. The correlation between the five genetic factors and the five normative factors taken from the NEO-PI-R manual was high at .83 (N), .72 (E), .92 (O), .88 (A), and .70 (C). This correspondence between the genetic and observed factor structures clearly suggests that all of the constituent parts within each broad domain share a common genetic basis that is independent of genetic factors that influence the other domains. Highly congruent genetic and phenotypic factor structures have been found among the scales of the CPI as well (Carey & DiLalla, 1994; Loehlin, 1982).

Moving to personality dysfunction, Livesley et al. (1998) extracted four highly congruent factors from the phenotypic, genetic, and environmental correlations computed between the eighteen DAPP dimensions. The DAPP was administered to three independent samples: 602 personality disordered nontwin patients, a general population sample of 939 nontwins, and general population sample of 686 twin pairs. The congruency coefficients ranged from .94 to .98. This analysis suggests that there are four basic personality disorders. The first is emotional dysregulation, which resembles Cluster B and the extreme aspects of neuroticism. The second is inhibition, which resembles Cluster C and the negative end of extraversion. The third is dissocial, which encompasses Cluster A and the negative extreme of agreeableness. The last is conscientiousness, which resembles the Cluster C obsessive-compulsive personality disorder diagnosis and the extreme end of conscientiousness.

As Widiger (1998, p. 865) put it, "Four out of five ain't bad." Only openness to experience does not appear to have a pathological extreme. This can be interpreted in three ways. First, extreme behaviors associated with this trait are not seen in clinical settings. This can mean that there are no negative consequences to being open-minded or willing to entertain new ideas. Second, it could mean that scales like the DAPP do not contain adequate content to measure these problems if they exist. Third, the status of openness as a bona fide personality trait is questionable. It has been argued that openness is simply cognitive ability or intelligence. However, this does not appear to be the case as the phenotypic and genetic correlations between measures of openness and cognitive ability have been shown to be quite small (e.g., Ashton, Lee, Vernon, & Jang, 2000).

ENVIRONMENTAL AND PSYCHOSOCIAL RISK FACTORS

Heritability analyses have consistently shown that nonshared environmental factors account for the majority of the individual differences in personality and its disorders. Multivariate genetic analyses have shown that these environmental influences are largely unique to each trait, and unlike genetic factors that tend to account for the covariation of traits, these environmental factors appear to play a role in differentiating traits. The next step is to identify what these environmental influences are.

The behavioral sciences have a long history of research on which environmental variables are important in personality development. Classic examples are birth order (Sulloway, 1995) and birth spacing (Zajonc, 1993). More recently, attention has been directed to the influence of peers over that of parents on adolescent development as described in Judith Harris' (1998) book *The Nurture Assumption*. The personality disorder literature has identified a number of risk factors, including dysfunctional families (e.g., the effects of parental psychopathology, family breakdown, pathogenic parenting practices), traumatic experiences (e.g., childhood sexual or physical abuse), and social stressors (reviewed in Paris, 2001). However, empirical research has shown that any one stressor accounts for a very small proportion of the variability in personality function. In fact, the clinical literature has consistently shown that there is no clear one-to-one association between early experience and the development of personality disorder (e.g., Garmezy & Masten, 1994; Rutter, 1989). Rather, adversities increase the eventual risk for mental disorders. Most people exposed to a particular risk factor do not develop any disorder, and people who develop a disorder may have been exposed to different risk factors.

This fact was highlighted by Turkheimer and Waldron (2000), whose extensive meta-analysis of all of the environmental research showed that studies assessing family constellation variables accounted for only 1.1% of the variance on average; differences in maternal and paternal behavior fared slightly better at 2.3% and 1.6%, respectively; differences in sibling interaction accounted for on average 4.1% and differences in peer-teacher interactions a sizeable 9.1% on average. They concluded that environmental effects must be cumulative—that it may take many such small effects to accumulate and have a measureable effect on behavior (p. 91). Another explanation for the small effect of individual environmental stressors is that the nonshared environment does not have much effect independent of preexisting genetic factors, and what is important is the interplay of genetic and environmental factors. The interplay of genetic and environmental factors should be thought of not only as increasing liability to disorder but also as providing protection from its development (Kendler & Eaves, 1986). This is often referred to as *resiliency*. A large body of research in developmental psychology has elucidated the precise mechanisms underlying resilience (e.g., Rutter, 1987, 1989, 2003). Studies of children at risk (e.g., Werner & Smith, 1992) have documented both biological and social aspects involved in developing some degree of "immunity" to adverse experiences.

Gene-Environment Correlation

The personality disorder literature frequently refers to "amplification" effects (Paris 1994, 1996). Amplification refers to the phenomenon where underlying genetic vulnerabilities are augmented by psychological and social factors to become overt disorder. This is a form of gene-environment correlation and there have been several reports of its importance to personality function. One of the first was Saudino, Pedersen, Lichtenstein, and McClearn's (1997) study, which showed that all of the genetic variability in controllable, desirable, and undesirable life events in women was common to the genetic influences underlying EPQ neuroticism and extraversion and NEO openness to experience. They also found that the heritable influences underlying personality had little influence on uncontrollable life events. This is not surprising because uncontrollable life events are by definition random and cannot be influenced by heritable factors.

Jang, Vernon, and Livesley (2000) conducted similar analyses between measures of the social environment of the family measured by the Family Environment Scale (FES: Moos & Moos, 1986) and personality disorder traits assessed by the DAPP. Significant genetic correlations were found between FES family cohesiveness and emotional dysregulation ($r_G = -.45$) and inhibition ($r_G = -.39$); FES family achievement orientation and dissocial behavior ($r_G = .38$), and inhibition ($r_G = -.58$); and FES family intellectual-cultural orientation and emotional dysregulation ($r_G = -.34$).

Gene-Environment Interaction and Personality Function

There have been several tests of gene-environment interaction effects on personality using adoption data. In this design the adopted children are classed as being genetically "high" or "low" on a given personality trait based on their biological parents' score. These children are then placed in adoptive homes that vary on a number of environmental variables. By measuring the home environment and the adopted children's behavior in these homes, it is a simple matter to compare children who were classified as genetically high and low on the personality trait to see if their behavior changes as a function of family environment.

Bergeman, Plomin, McClearn, Pedersen, and Friberg (1988) found that adopted-away twins genetically low on extraversion who were placed in homes low in family control, family organization, and system maintenance (as measured by the FES) had higher extraversion scores compared to twins placed in adoptive homes high on these dimensions. In contrast, these variables did not influence twins who were high on extraversion. The same genotype-environmental interaction was also found for neuroticism, but in this case the active environmental agent was parental socioeconomic status. In other studies (Cadoret, Winokur, Langbehn, & Troughton, 1996; Cadoret, Yates, Troughton, Woodworth, & Stewart, 1995), adverse home environments were found to increase symptoms of conduct disorder and aggression only among adoptees who were at high genetic risk for conduct disorder (their biological parents scored high for antisocial personality).

Recently, Riggins-Capser et al. (1999) showed that what the adoptive parents know about the biological parents of their adopted children can also lead to clear gene-environment interaction effects. Information about biological parents is sometimes released depending on the adoption agency. The adoptive families were split into three groups: (a) were told nothing and had no knowledge, (b) knew physical characteristics of the biological parents such as height and weight, and (c) had knowledge of the psychiatric and medical background of the biological parents because they were told about psychological problems, alcoholism, and drug use.

The adoptive children were assessed for antisocial personality and split into two groups of genetically high or low, based on the biological parents' background. Clear interactions were detected. Levels of aggression, conduct disorder, and ADHD in the adopted children varied as a function of how much the adoptive parents knew about their adopted childrens' biological parents. The data showed that the behavioral differences between adopted children classified as genetically high or low on a behavioral measure are much smaller in families that know nothing about the biological parents' physical or health status.

One of the most dramatic examples of gene-environment interaction is the study by Caspi, McClay, and Moffitt (2002) on the development of antisocial behavior. They noted that one major risk factor for the development of antisocial behavior in boys (identified in clinical research) is abuse as a child, specifically erratic, coercive, and punitive parenting. As previously noted, there is little one-to-one correspondence between environmental factors and the development of disorder and the precipitant is whether the child has inherited a genetic liability. In the case of antisocial behavior, the monoamine oxidase A gene (MAOA gene) was selected because it has been associated with aggressive behavior in mice and in some studies of humans.

Caspi et al.'s (2002) sample consisted of 1,037 children who had been assessed at nine different ages for levels of maltreatment (no maltreatment, probable maltreatment, and severe maltreatment) and MAOA activity (low or high activity). They found that the effect of maltreatment was significantly weaker among males with high MAOA activity than those with low MAOA activity. Moreover, the probable and high maltreatment groups did not differ in MAOA activity, indicating that the genotype did not influence exposure to maltreatment. These results demonstrate that the MAOA gene modifies the influence of maltreatment.

THE GENES FOR PERSONALITY

The last study highlighted the importance of specific genes in the development of behavior. Molecular genetic research on personality is an extremely active area of research pioneered by Robert Cloninger (1986) and his Psychobiological Model of Temperament and Character, which has guided the selection of candidate genes in the past decade. This model hypothesizes that personality is composed of four temperament traits and three character traits. The temperament traits manifest early in life, functioning as preconceptual biases in perceptual memory and habit formation. Each trait is hypothesized to be controlled by a unique genetically based neurotransmitter system: the dopaminergic system for novelty seeking (NS); the serotonergic system for harm avoidance (HA); and the noradrenergic system for reward dependence (RD). A fourth dimension, persistence (P), has also been suggested (Cloninger et al., 1993), but no corresponding neurotransmitter system has yet been hypothesized.

The three character dimensions are self-directedness (SD), cooperativeness (CO), and self-transcendence (ST), which are hypothesized to be traits that reflect learned, maturational variations in goals, values, and self-concepts that develop in adulthood through conceptual or insight-based learning. As such, the character traits should show little heritable influence in contrast to the temperament traits.

Dopamine and Novelty Seeking

The first successful study in the search for personality genes was that of Cloninger et al.'s (1996), who reported an association between novelty seeking and the dopamine receptor DRD4. The DRD4 gene is known to exist in a short and a long form. The shorter alleles code for a receptor that is more efficient in binding dopamine, whereas the long form of the allele is less efficient. Cloninger et al. hypothesized that individuals with the long DRD4 allele are dopamine deficient and seek novelty to increase dopamine release. In support of the psychobiological model, novelty-seeking scores of individuals with the long form of the allele were significantly higher than those of individuals with the short form of the allele.

After the euphoria and media frenzy that accompanied this report, several independent laboratories were able to replicate this association (e.g., Benjamin, Greenberg, & Murphy, 1996; Ebstein, Novick, & Umansky, 1996; Ebstein, Segman, & Benjamin, 1997). However, there have been as many failures to replicate the association (e.g., Ebstein, Gritsenko, & Nemanov, 1997; Gebhardt et al., 1997; Malhotra, Goldman, Ozaki, & Breier, 1996; Ono et al., 1999; Pogue-Geile, Ferrell, Deka, Debski, & Manuck, 1998; Vandenbergh, Zonderman, Wang, Uhl, & Costa, 1997). Moreover, it is important to note that among the successful replications, the DRD4 gene accounted for only a very small proportion of the variance in novelty seeking (approximately 5%). This suggests that although the DRD4 allele does contributes to novelty seeking, its effect is very small.

Another reason for the inconsistent results is that Cloninger's (1994) scale (the Tridimensional Personality Questionnaire [TPQ] and its present incarnation the TCI) has been criticized for a number of psychometric and conceptual problems that could have reduced the power to detect an association. De Fruyt, van de Wiele, and van Heeringen (2000) correlated the TPQ with the NEO-PI-R and showed that, although much of the content of the TPQ is related to the Big Five personality dimensions in predictable ways, the scales were unexpectedly related to other dimensions. For example, TPQ novelty seeking was positively related to extraversion but also found to be negatively related to conscientiousness.

The psychometric problems with Cloninger's (1994) scales may also contribute to the equivocal heritability estimates found for this measure. For example, on a sample of 296 twin pairs from Japan (184 MZ and 112 DZ pairs), Ando et al. (2002) showed that either additive genetic (h^2_A) or common environmental effects (c^2) could explain the variance on novelty seeking and reward dependence. Thus, it comes as no surprise that the genotyping results have been extremely difficult to replicate. Considering these problems, several labs have used other measures with well-established psychometric properties such as the NEO-PI-R instead. Another trend has been to examine other dopaminergic genes such as the dopamine D2 receptor (DRD2).

Sadly, the switch to different measures and candidate genes continues to produce conflicting results. For example, Burt, McGue, Iacono, Comings, and MacMurray (2002) reported no association between DRD4 or the DRD2 and novelty seeking measured by the MPQ using data from 137 families from the Minnesota Twin Family Study. In contrast, Berman, Ozkaragoz, Young, and Noble (2002) reported a positive association between the DRD2 and TPQ novelty seeking in a study of 203 adolescent males.

Neuroticism and Serotonin

Another line of research centers on neuroticism. Instead of relying on a theoretical model like Cloninger's psychobiological model (1993) to guide the selection of candidate genes, researchers have turned to empirical studies of humans and primates that demonstrate that levels of specific neurotransmitters actually do influence behavior. For example, Knutson et al. (1998) found that administration of paroxetine, a specific serotonin reuptake inhibitor that targets the serotonin transporter, both decreased negative affect and increased scores on a behavioral index of social affiliation in normal human subjects.

This type of clinical finding has led researchers to associate serotonin polymorphisms with neuroticism. Like the DRD4, the expression of the human serotonin transporter gene 5-HTTLPR exists in long and short forms. The short form of this allele is dominant to the long version, with the long version of the 5-HTTLPR genotype producing more serotonin transporter mRNA and protein than the short form in cultured cells, platelets, and brain tissue. Results have shown that individuals possessing the short form of the allele have significantly increased NEO-PI-R scores (e.g., Lesch et al., 1996) and related traits such as harm avoidance as measured by the TPQ (e.g., Katsuragi et al., 1999). More interestingly, Hamer and colleagues (1999) found associations between the "learned" character traits of cooperativeness and self-directedness and the 5-HTTLPR. This association questions the distinction between heritable temperament and nonheritable character.

Despite these successes, a number of studies have not found an association between the serotonin transporter and either NEO-PI-R neuroticism (Gelernter, Kranzler, Coccaro, Siever, & New, 1998) or TPQ harm avoidance (Hamer, Greenberg, Sabol, & Murphy, 1999). A recent study by Hariri, Mattay, and Tessitore (2002) also did not find a significant association between harm avoidance and the serotonin transporter. However, they did find a significant association between the serotonin transporter and neurotic behavior, specifically, anxiety and fear, and found that it was also associated with greater neuronal activity in the amygdala. Specifically, they showed that individuals who possessed the short form of the allele had lower 5-HT function and expression, relatively higher levels of synaptic 5-HT and expression, and greater activity in the amygdala when matching affect-laden stimuli (matching angry or fearful faces to a target) than individuals who were homozygous for the long form of the allele. The significance of this study once again highlights the importance of selecting the correct phenotype.

Bigger, Faster, Better

It can be argued that molecular genetic research is limited by traditional self-report personality assessments that are of little value, and that endophenotypic personality measurements must be developed. The reality is that personality researchers will depend on paper-and-pencil personality scales for the foreseeable future. The question is how research designs can be modified to take advantage of their best features but at the same time ameliorate or circumvent their liabilities? One general approach is to design a more powerful study.

Plomin et al. (2003) outlined several design features for molecular genetic studies to increase their power to reliably detect genes. Some ideas include undertaking large, longitudinal population-based studies, conducting genome scans using more markers, and identifying better candidate genes to reduce genotyping error. These approaches tend to rely on brute force to overcome error. A second approach is to create genetically indexed measures of personality. Sham et al. (2000) recently described a basic process that enables a score on any measure to be split in half. One score reflects the influence of genetic factors and the other the environmental influence. It is theoretically possible to divide the genetic score further to reflect the variability in neuroticism due to specific alleles like 5-HTTLPR or DRD4. These genetically and environmentally indexed scales would reduce environmental and genetic variation on a behavioral measure that is not associated with the putative loci and would increase the power to find them (Lander & Botstein, 1989). For clinicians, such scales would be extremely useful as they could index and identify the differential effects of psychotherapeutic or pharmacological treatments by tracking changes in the environmental or genetic scores.

One way to develop these scores is to derive a weight for each of the genetic and environmental effects that can be applied to the score of a questionnaire. These weights can be thought of as regression weights, but rather than being derived from the phenotypic correlations between a set of variables, they are instead derived from a set of genetic (r_G) and environmental correlations (r_E). For example, imagine that a matrix of genetic correlations is subjected to a factor analysis and two nonoverlapping factors are extracted. A score for each person on each of the factors can be computed by multiplying each person's response to each item by a weight that reflects only the genetic effects attributable to that factor (Fig. 5.5). The same procedure can be applied to the environmental correlations to derive scores that reflect only the environmental influences unique to that factor.

The value of genetic and environmental scores over the phenotypic scores in genotyping studies has been demonstrated in several simulation studies and in studies using actual data (Cardon et al., 1994; Eaves & Meyer, 1994). Boomsma (1996) reported a two-fold increase in power to detect linkage using squared differences of individual genetic factor scores compared with squared differences of phenotypic scores between pairs of siblings.

SUMMARY

In this chapter I discussed the behavioral genetic research that has had a bearing on three central issues in personality disorder research: (a) the validity of the dimensional model of personality and its disorders, (b) the definition of the major personality domains, and (c) the number of personality diagnoses. Behavioral genetic research has shown that virtually all measures of normal and abnormal personality are heritable to about the same degree. Additive genetic effects account for 40% to 45%, and nonshared environmental factors account for the remainder. These estimates are extremely stable and have been replicated across several twin studies

---

$$y = \gamma \Sigma^{-1} x$$

Where y = factor score for the common genetic factor, γ = the factor loadings of each variable on the genetic factor of interest (i.e., the column vector of estimated path coefficients, which represent the correlations between the common genetic or environmental factor and the observed measures), Σ^{-1} = correlation matrix between all of the variables (i.e., the inverse of the correlation matrix of the observed measures), and x = each person's score or response to each of the variables (i.e., column vector of observed values on the measures).

FIG. 5.5. A method that permits the computation of genetic factor scores.

worldwide. Multivariate genetic research has shown that measures of normal and abnormal personality share a common genetic basis, supporting the validity of the dimensional model. Environmental influences have been found to be largely specific to measures of personality, suggesting that these factors differentiate normal and abnormal behavior. The identification of these factors and action mechanisms are presently the focus of intense investigation.

Although personality researchers have come to a general consensus that personality can be adequately described by five broad domains (neuroticism, extraversion, openness to experience, agreeableness, and conscientiousness), questions remain regarding the subtraits defining each domain. For example, all measures of extraversion recognize sociability and affiliation, but not all incorporate agency (e.g., surgency, exhibitionism), activation (e.g., activity level), impulsivity or sensation seeking, positive emotions, or optimism. Similarly, questions remain about whether impulsivity should be a component of neuroticism. Multivariate genetic models have examined this issue by testing whether all subtraits defining a domain share a common genetic basis. It has generally been found that each domain is composed of two genetically unique clusters of subtraits that overlap to some degree. These models suggest that broad domains of personality are not inherited, but are rather trait clusters with a common genetic basis. The domains appear to be a convenient way to reflect the common genetic basis of traits.

Multivariate genetic analyses have extracted four highly congruent phenotypic, genetic, and environmental factors of personality dysfunction: emotional dysregulation (resembling Cluster B personality disorders and the extreme aspects of neuroticism), inhibition (resembling Cluster C personality disorders and the negative end of extraversion), antisocial (encompassing the Cluster A personality disorders and the negative extreme of agreeableness), and conscientiousness (resembling the Cluster C obsessive compulsive personality disorder diagnosis and the extreme end of conscientiousness). Only openness to experience does not appear to have a pathological extreme. This is because extreme behaviors associated with this trait are not seen in clinical settings. The fact that these four factors have been found in patient and general population samples further supports the dimensional model of personality disorder.

Chapter 6

The Anxiety Disorders

Psychotherapy involves unlearning, learning, and relearning. The patient must learn how to undo old maladaptive patterns (unlearning), develop new and more effective coping mechanisms (learning), and then reinforce these new patterns of behavior by repetition (relearning).

—John Ogrodniczuk (personal communication, 2004)

The opening quotation was taken from a colleague's lecture on the mechanisms of psychotherapy to highlight a theme of this chapter—the role of learning in the development and treatment of mental disorder. An idea that has emerged from the behavioral genetic literature on the anxiety disorders is that different learning processes are a significant source of shared and nonshared environmental influences. This idea is the result of the clinical treatment literature showing that behavioral therapies are among the most effective means to treat these disorders (e.g., Nathan & Gorman, 2002) coupled with the fact that many of the anxiety disorders have been consistently shown to be among the most influenced by shared (c^2) and nonshared (e^2) environmental factors of the common disorders.

Three kinds of learning are thought to be important in the initiation, shaping, and maintenance of psychopathology: classical conditioning, operant conditioning, and social or observational learning. Classical conditioning is the pairing of behavior with random benign or aversive stimuli. The best known example is Pavlov's experiment with dogs, in which the anticipation of food (indexed by salivation) was paired with the sound of a bell. Operant conditioning is the process by which behavior is shaped—for example, teaching a dove to turn a pirouette by rewarding movement of its feet in the correct directions and punishing movement in the wrong direction. Social or observational learning (e.g., Bandura, 1986) posits that behavior is acquired from the observation of other people, such as family members.

In behavioral genetics, the process of learning is often overlooked as an important source of shared and nonshared environmental influence because most attention is paid to objective aspects of the environment (e.g., the actual number of stressors in the workplace, levels of family support, or strictness of teachers). Learning as a source of environmental effect, however, is readily integrated into quantitative genetic theory. For example, if behavior was acquired solely by learning, h^2 would equal zero and c^2 and e^2 effects would account for all of the variability. However, to put a finer point on it, if the primary learning process was social or observational learning, c^2 would account for more variability than e^2 because the learning environment is shared by all members of a family living in the same home. On the other hand, if the primary learning process was classical conditioning, c^2 would equal zero with e^2 accounting for all of the variability because the learning occurred solely as a result of experiences that are unique to each individual. If operant conditioning was the primary means behavior was acquired, behavioral genetic theory predicts that e^2 would account for more than c^2. Avoidance learning, for example, is usually the product of experiencing some kind of unique aversive event (e.g., being bitten by a snake) but it can also be the product of observational learning in the home (e.g., mother displayed fear when spotting a snake in the garden).

All learning begins with some form of preexisting behavior common to all members of a species. Teaching a dove to turn a pirouette can only be accomplished because the bird is able to move its feet to the left or right. This last point is particularly important. If we extrapolate to human behavior; this model demands that psychopathology must have a basis in normal behavior; for example, a phobia develops from a normal fear response. Multivariate genetic models investigating whether normal fear and phobia share a common genetic and environmental basis provide a test of this hypothesis.

The chapter is organized into three broad sections. The first reviews heritability studies of the anxiety disorder diagnoses. Estimates of h^2, c^2, and e^2 and the degree to which the diagnoses share these influences are reviewed. The second section discusses research on the premorbid forms of these disorders by examining the evidence that the anxiety disorders are extreme forms of normal-range behavior. The last section examines research that attempts to integrate learning, genetics, and the environment into a comprehensive model of how psychopathology can develop.

HERITABILITY OF THE ANXIETY DISORDER DIAGNOSES

Most of the behavioral genetic literature has focused on panic disorder, posttraumatic stress disorder (PTSD), obsessive-compulsive disorder (OCD), generalized anxiety disorder (GAD), and the phobias (including social phobia, blood and injury phobia, and agoraphobia). A recent meta-analysis of published twin, family, and adoption studies indicated that these diagnoses were all moderately familial and heritable (Hettema, Neale, & Kendler, 2001). The morbidity risk for OCD, panic, GAD, and the phobias were estimated to range between 0.7% and 11.7%; 7.9% and 17.3%; 8.9% and 19.7%; and 10.0% and 26.4%, respectively. The twin studies estimated the heritability (h^2_B) of panic disorder to range between 37% and 43%, with e^2 comprising the remainder. The heritability of GAD was estimated at $h^2_B = 22\%-37\%$, $c^2 = 17\%-25\%$, and e^2 comprised the remainder. The heritability of the phobias was similar at $h^2_B = 20\%-39\%$, $c^2 = 27\%-32\%$, and $e^2 = 61\%-80\%$.

Meta-analyses like these are popular because they permit conclusions to be drawn across several studies. However, it is important to remember that the rigor with which they summarize research can be a double-edged sword. First, it is very easy to exclude high-quality studies if there are too many inclusion criteria. Second, effect sizes can be inflated because often only studies that report significant effects are published. Third, excellent studies may be excluded because they are published in journals that are difficult to access (e.g., due to language, availability at a university library, or absence from a publication database like PsychINFO or MedLine). With this in mind, the following subsections provide a wider review of the most recent heritability studies to round out the aetiological picture.

Panic Disorder

Twin Studies. One of the most interesting twin studies of panic was that of Kendler, Neale, Kessler, Heath, and Eaves' (1993), which showed that when trained clinicians made the diagnosis, panic disorder was significantly heritable. However, when a computer algorithm that rigorously applied the diagnostic rules made the diagnosis, h^2 dropped to 0.0%! These estimates were based on a sample of 236 general population female twin pairs who met *DSM-III-R* (1987) criteria for panic disorder. The twins were assigned to one of three categories: "definite" in which all criteria were met; "possible" where there was some modest uncertainty about some criteria but the diagnosis was deemed appropriate; and "probable," or cases that clinically appeared to have a psychiatric disorder closely resembling panic disorder but did not meet full criteria. A total of 126 pairs met the criteria for a "definite" diagnosis, whereas the remaining 110 were labeled as "probable." Given these relatively small sample sizes, they combined the "definite" and "probable" groups into a single category called "narrow panic disorder" and the other into the category "broad panic disorder."

The heritability (h^2_A) of narrow panic disorder was 46%, $c^2 = 0.0\%$, $e^2 = 54\%$ by clinician rating but by computer algorithm $h^2_A = 0.0\%$, $c^2 = 32\%$, $e^2 = 68\%$. In contrast, for broad panic disorder the estimates on clinician and computer assignments were similar: by clinician $h^2_A = 32\%$, $c^2 = 0.0\%$, $e^2 = 68\%$ and by computer algorithm $h^2_A = 37\%$, $c^2 = 0.0\%$, $e^2 = 63\%$. They felt that the results from the computer-based application were likely anomalous because computers do not have the benefit of any additional written information from clinical interview, which limits the validity of blind and mechanistic application of criteria. Alternatively, it could mean that what is heritable is not the patient's actual condition but the clinician's ability to make a diagnosis.

Of particular interest in this study was the finding that shared family influences (c^2) was zero. This finding was significant because it eliminated the role of social learning in the aetiology of this disorder. This finding was replicated in a later study by Kendler et al. (1995), who not only measured panic quantitatively to take advantage of the greater variability in the data, but also analyzed data from the twins' parents (where available), which permitted a direct estimation of c^2 effects.

Panic was assessed using thirty items from the self-report ninety-item Symptom Check List (SCL-90: Derogatis, 1994). Twins for this paper came from two sources: the population-based Virginia Twin Registry and self-selected twins recruited through the American Association of Retired Persons (AARP). The thirty items were factored and a "Panic-Phobia" primary factor was extracted, which was defined by high loadings from items assessing spells of terror and panic as well as by a large number of items assessing phobic symptoms, in particular, symptoms of agoraphobia, such as fear of travel, sudden fear, avoidance of frightening things, and fear of being alone. This factor is interesting because it suggests that symptoms of panic and phobia are not independent of one another as is currently assumed. The heritability of the panic-phobia factor in the general population sample was 47.1% for males and 29.8% for females; in the AARP sample, the broad heritability was estimated at 72.9% for males and 24.0% for females. No c^2 effects were found in either sample. Of interest is the finding that heritability of the AARP males is much greater. The authors suggested that this is due to greater volunteer bias in the AARP sample, but the heritable nature of this disorder was still confirmed.

Molecular Genetic Studies Of Panic.   Assuming that panic disorder has a significant heritable basis, several molecular genetic studies have been undertaken to identify possible susceptibility genes, but the results have been mixed. Hamilton et al. (1999) genotyped 340 individuals from the families of 45 panic disorder probands and found no differences in allele frequencies or linkage to the serotonin transporter (5-HTT). The null results were found despite testing several models of inheritance that specified different degrees of genetic dominance and recessiveness. Similarly, little has been found in the dopaminergic system. On a sample of 622 individuals from 70 proband families with panic disorder, Hamilton et al. (2000) found no association or linkage with the D4 dopamine receptor (DRD4) or the dopamine transporter (DAT).

Some positive linkages have been found between the serotonin receptor ($5HT_{2A}R$) gene on chromosome 13 and "panic syndrome," as opposed to a strict diagnosis of panic disorder (Weissman et al., 2000). The panic syndrome used in this study encompassed the usual diagnostic criteria for panic disorder, but was broadened to include the primary physical complaints associated with the disorder such as kidney and bladder problems, serious headaches, thyroid problems (usually hypothyroidism), and mitral valve prolapses. With this broadened definition they found significant linkage (l.o.d. score = 3.2) in families with panic disorder and specifically bladder or kidney problems, but no linkage was found in families when only panic disorder but no physical complaints were analyzed. These findings suggest that there is a separation between psychological and physical symptoms where the somatic complaints might be accounting for the inherited or genetic aspects of the disorder, whereas the mental symptoms are a product of learning. This apparent separation of physical and mental symptoms has been seen with other disorders such as the mood disorders discussed in chapter 4.

Generalized Anxiety Disorder

Several twin studies have shown that Generalized Anxiety Disorder (GAD) is heritable. For example, Kendler, Neale, Kessler, Heath, and Eaves (1992c) estimated h^2 at 33%, and recent studies have shown that the genetic factors influencing males were the same as those influencing females (Hettema et al., 2001). The big question regarding GAD is not whether it is heritable, but rather whether it should continue to be recognized as a distinct disorder, given that anxiety is a symptom found in most, if not all, of the common disorders. The presence of anxiety in most disorders has led some to wonder if GAD might actually be a broad liability to mental disorder and if it might best be used as a marker for people at risk for developing future disorder. Multivariate genetic analyses have yet to provide a clear answer.

A family study by Noyes, Clarkson, Crowe, Yates, and McChesney (1987) supports the differentiation of GAD from panic disorder defined by *DSM-III-R* (1987) criteria. They found that the frequency of GAD was higher among first-degree relatives of probands with GAD (19.5%) than among relatives of healthy controls (3.5%), demonstrating that GAD is familial. However, GAD was not found at a higher rate among first-degree relatives of probands with a primary diagnosis of panic disorder (5.4%) or agoraphobia (3.9%), suggesting that GAD is a separate entity. This study is notable in that it outlined clinical features shared by GAD probands and their first-degree relatives. This information is important for counseling family of an affected individual on their risk of developing GAD. The symptoms shared were: anxious expectation, vigilance and scanning, motor tension, and autonomic hyperactivity. However, relatives of GAD probands were older at onset and had a significantly shorter median duration of illness. They report that more of the relatives went into remission, but fewer had secondary depression and abnormal personality traits. In contrast, Kendler, Neale, Kessler, Heath, and Eaves (1992c, 1992d) demonstrated that the genetic factors underlying *DSM-III-R* GAD could only be explained during comorbid episodes of panic disorder or lifetime major depression. These findings were later replicated in males and females using twin data from Sweden (Roy, Neale, Pedersen, Mathé, & Kendler, 1995) and what appears to differentiate GAD from other disorders such as major depression is exposure to specific environmental influences. Roy et al. (p. 1046) reported that major depression is related predominantly to "loss events," including death of a relative or loss of a job, whereas GAD is related mainly to "danger events" such as events "that might elicit future crisis." However, they also noted that the environmental risk factors for each disorder are not 100% independent.

The Phobias

The meta-analysis presented earlier suggested that the phobias are modestly heritable, ranging from 20% to 39% (Hettema, Neale, & Kendler, 2001). Not apparent from this meta-analysis is that some phobias are differentially and highly heritable. For example, Kendler, Karkowski, and Prescott (1999) reported the heritability of *DSM-III* blood or injury phobia at 60%, 50% for situational phobia, and 50% for social phobia. Agoraphobia was highly heritable but attributable to nonadditive genetic effects (h^2_d = 61%). For animal phobia, they modified the definition to include or exclude the "unreasonable fears" criterion. When the definition excluded unreasonable fears, animal phobia (e.g., avoidance behavior, intense anxiety response) was not heritable at all. When unreasonable fears were included in the definition, h^2_A went to 47% and c^2 dropped to 0.00%. They suggested that the "unreasonable fear" of animals is the heritable component of the phobias because it is innate, possibly an artifact of early human evolutionary history when avoiding animals conferred real advantages for survival and reproduction.

The substantial heritable basis of the phobias suggests that they share a common genetic basis. This was confirmed by Kendler, Neale, Kessler, Heath, and Eaves (1993) who found that an independent pathways model specifying one common additive genetic but also one common nonshared environmental factor explained the covariance of *DSM-III* (1980) agoraphobia, and social, situational, and simple phobias in 2,163 general population female twins.

The overall heritability of agoraphobia, and social, animal, and situational phobias was 36%, 35%, 35%, and 29%. However, the common genetic factor accounted for 7%, 10%, 35%, and 9% of the total variance in each, whereas the common environmental factor accounted for 64%, 32%, 5%, and 17% in these diagnoses. Genetic factors unique to agoraphobia accounted for 29% of the total variance, and other unique factors were 21% for social phobia, 0% for animal phobia, and 20% for situational phobia.

These findings show that the phobias share a common aetiological basis, but are influenced to a significant degree by genetic and environmental factors unique to each. These findings are important because they challenge popular ideas about this disorder. There is one school of thought that suggests that the phobias are qualitatively different from each other. For example, each phobia must represent an independent disorder because the phobic stimuli for social phobia or agoraphobia, for example, are relatively diffuse compared to those for the animal phobias, which are well circumscribed. However, the finding that the phobias share to a significant degree a common aetiological basis does not entirely support this idea. Moreover, the results do not support the alternative view that each of the different phobias are no more than minor variations of a broader construct because the analyses have shown that the vast majority of the genetic variability on agoraphobia and simple phobia for example, come from genetic factors unique to each. Rather, Kendler et al. (1993), noted that their results fall halfway between these two extreme theoretical models. They suggested that the relationship between the different phobia types are best understood if they are ordered along a genetic continuum bounded at one end by agoraphobia (which derives the least of its genetic variability from the common factor) and at the other end simple phobias (which derive most of their genetic variance from the source common to all).

Social phobia deserves special attention because of questions regarding its relationship to avoidant personality disorder (APD). The symptoms of both disorders are phenotypically similar and are frequently comorbid (e.g., Jansen, Arntz, Merckelbach, & Mersch, 1994), raising the question of whether APD is really a personality disorder or just an extreme case of social phobia. A family study of *DSM-IV* (1994) generalized social phobia and APD suggests the latter. Stein, Chartier, Hazen, et al. (1998) assessed two types of social phobia by direct interview. The first was "generalized social phobia," defined as pervasive, debilitating social phobia of the type usually seen in patients. The second was "nongeneralized social phobia," the fear of one or two circumscribed situations, such as public speaking. They found that the relative risk for generalized social phobia and APD was ten times higher among first-degree relatives of patients with generalized social phobia. In contrast, the relative risk for nongeneralized social phobia was not significantly different, suggesting that only generalized social phobia is familial, and that APD may be an extreme form of generalized social phobia.

The consistent heritable and familial basis of social phobia has prompted several attempts to identify the putative loci. Stein, Chartier, Kozak, King, and Kennedy (1998) conducted one of the first studies of the serotonin transporter (5-HTT) gene located on chromosome 17 and the serotonin receptor ($5HT_{2A}R$) gene located on chromosome 13. These genes were chosen for several reasons. First, social phobia has been shown to be responsive to selective serotonin reuptake inhibitors (SSRIs) that cause changes in the 5-HTT gene. Second, generalized social phobia is frequently comorbid with MDD, panic disorder, and OCD, all of which have been the focus of intensive study via the serotonin system (e.g., McDougle, Epperson, Price & Gelernter, 1998). Third, social phobics have elevated scores on harm avoidance that have been associated with $5HT_{2A}R$ binding to blood platelets (Nelson, Cloninger, Przybeck, & Csernansky, 1996). Sadly, despite the strong a priori reasons to focus on the serotonergic system, no linkages were detected using *DSM-IV* (1994) criteria for social phobia (26 subjects), generalized social phobia (13 subjects), or APD (37 subjects).

Obsessive-Compulsive Disorder

There is a great deal of research that has demonstrated that OCD runs in families. For example, Black, Goldstein, Noyes, and Blum (1995) reported that the risk for OCD was higher for parents of obsessional probands than parents of controls (16% vs. 3%). However, more recent research has shown that obsessive and compulsive symptoms stem from different genetically based systems. Nestdadt et al. (2000) conducted a blind, controlled family study of OCD by comparing rates of the disorder in 80 probands and 343 first-degree relatives to 73 control probands and 300 of their first-degree relatives to establish the familiality of the disorder. Lifetime prevalence of OCD was significantly higher in case than in control relatives (11.7% vs. 2.7%) and age of onset also had a familial basis—no symptoms were detected in relatives of probands whose age at onset was 18 years or older. However, they also found that only the rate of obsessive symptomology was higher in case relatives, suggesting obsessions and compulsions are influenced by different aetiological factors. Jonnal, Garnder, Prescott, and Kendler (2000) reported a similar result. They administered a twenty-item self-report measure of OCD symptoms to 527 twin pairs from Virginia. Two factors were extracted: The first described obsessions and the second described compulsions. Heritability analyses estimated h^2_A at 33% and 26%, respectively, and the genetic correlation (r_G) between the factors was .53, suggesting that obsessions and compulsions only partially stem from the same genetic causes. Interestingly, they also found that probands with tics or obsessive-compulsive personality disorder (OCPD) were not more likely to have relatives with OCD than those without these features. This result is important as it suggests that OCD and OCPD are aetiologically distinct disorders.

OCD is also frequently comorbid with Gilles de la Tourette's Syndrome (TS) and evidence from family studies suggests they also share a common aetiological basis. Pauls, Alsobrook, Goodman, Rasmussen, and Leckman (1995) compared the rates of OCD, TS, and chronic tics in 466 first-degree relatives of 100 probands diagnosed with OCD to 33 controls and 113 of their first-degree relatives. The rate of OCD (10.3%) and subthreshold OCD (7.9%) was significantly higher in relatives of probands with OCD than relatives of normal healthy controls (1.9% and 2.0%, respectively). Furthermore, the rate of TS and chronic tics was greater in relatives of OCD probands (4.6%) than the control relatives (1.0%).

In contrast to adult forms of OCD, Reddy et al. (2001) reported on the rates of juvenile OCD and TS in first-degree relatives of 35 OCD probands (*DSM-III-R*, 1987, criteria) aged 16 years or younger compared to 34 matched control cases and their first-degree relatives. The morbid risk for juvenile OCD among relatives of juvenile OCD probands was a low 4.96%, whereas no cases of juvenile OCD were found among the first-degree relatives. Moreover, they did not find any cases of TS or other tic disorder in any of the relatives of juvenile OCD probands or the control subjects, suggesting that most cases of juvenile OCD are nonfamilial and unrelated to the tic disorders. The finding that juvenile OCD is not familial stands in contrast to the adult forms of the disorder, which is at least moderately heritable, suggesting, as had the Nestdadt et al. (2000) study, that the familial liability is age related.

Besides TS, OCD is frequently comorbid with other disorders and the basis of the comorbidity has been the subject of a great deal of behavioral genetic research. For example, Nestdadt et al. (2001) examined the familial relationship between OCD, anxiety, and affective disorders. In general, all anxiety and affective disorders (except bipolar disorder) were ascertained more frequently in case than in control probands. Specifically, GAD, panic disorder, agoraphobia, separation anxiety disorder, and recurrent major depression were more common in case than control relatives. Interestingly, the rates of panic disorder, separation anxiety disorder, and recurrent major depression only occurred more frequently if the relative was also diagnosed with OCD, suggesting that anxiety and affective disorders, when comorbid with OCD, may have developed as a consequence of the OCD. Because GAD and agoraphobia were more frequent in case relatives independent of OCD, the authors suggested that GAD and agoraphobia share in part a common familial aetiology with OCD.

Bienvenu et al. (2000) examined the relationship between OCD and "obsessive-compulsive" spectrum disorders, such as somatoform disorders (body dysmorphic disorder and hypochondriasis), the eating disorders (anorexia and bulimia nervosa), impulse-control disorders (e.g., kleptomania, pathological gambling, pyromania), and pathological "grooming" conditions (nail biting, skin picking, trichotillomania) using *DSM-IV* (1994) criteria. They found that body dysmorphic disorder, hypochondriasis, and any eating or grooming disorder occurred more frequently in case probands. In addition, either somatoform disorder or a grooming condition occurred more frequently in case relatives, regardless of whether the case probands had the same diagnosis. The findings suggest that certain somatoform or pathological grooming conditions are part of a familial OCD spectrum. Though other spectrum conditions may resemble OCD, they do not appear to be important aspects of the familial spectrum.

Posttraumatic Stress Disorder

The literature contains several heritability studies of posttraumatic stress disorder (PTSD) because of the availability of large numbers of twins involved in combat in the Vietnam War. PTSD is unique among anxiety disorders in that it is defined in the context of exposure to an extremely stressful and circumscribed traumatic event. Accordingly, there has been as much focus on risk factors for experiencing these events as on the resulting symptomology.

True et al. (1993) surveyed 2,224 MZ and 1,818 DZ pairs on fifteen PTSD symptoms taken from the three symptom clusters in the *DSM-III* (1980) and *DSM-III-R* (1987): (a) Traumatic events are persistently reexperienced, (b) persistent avoidance of stimuli associated with trauma or numbing of general responsiveness, and (c) persistent symptoms of increased arousal. The twins were split into two groups: those who had served in Southeast Asia (SEA) and those who had not. The first set of heritability analyses focused on the twins who had not served in SEA. This analysis is important because the results obtained from these veterans would be the most applicable to the general population. The heritability (h^2_B) of all fifteen symptoms was very similar, ranging from 32% to 45%. When the data from the twins who had served in SEA was added, estimates did not change significantly, indicating that differences in trauma exposure did not mediate genetic control of the resulting symptomology. It also showed that responses to trauma did not depend on the type of event experienced and that PTSD is not a disorder solely associated with military service.

The heritability of PTSD has left some wondering how to identify individuals with a high genetic liability for that disorder (e.g., via blood test), for whom the risk of exposure to traumatic events could be limited (e.g., assigning new military recruits to noncombat duties). Radant, Tsuang, Peskind, McFall, and Raskind (2001) suggested that hypothalamic-pituitary-adrenal axis (the HPA axis is a major part of the neuroendocrine system that controls reaction to stress) hypofunction, physiologic markers of increased arousal, and increased acoustic startle response are all potential PTSD markers. Some work has been done in this area using animal models. For example, King, Abend, and Edwards (2001) discussed a variant of the classic learned helplessness model (Seligman, 1971), called the "congenital learned helplessness model" (cLH). This model focuses on changes in biologically based responses (e.g., pain tolerance, spatial memory, HPA functioning) to intermittent stress in the presence and absence of situational cues. They found that animals in the cLH condition displayed increased pain tolerance and 80% of the animals displayed a decrease in performance on spatial memory tests and blunted poststress corticosterone response (corticosterone is an immune hormone whose level is a major indicator of stress), suggesting they are valuable markers of PTSD-proneness.

Despite the heritable basis of PTSD, environmental effects remain the most important factor in its development. King, King, Foy, Keane, and Fairbank (1999) examined data from 432 female and 1,200 male veterans of the Vietnam War to identify specific environmental factors that have a causal relationship to PTSD. They conducted extensive interviews of the veterans and collected data on prewar background and functioning, military and war zone experiences, postwar circumstances, life events, and mental health status. They conducted analyses for women and men separately. For women, the following variables had a positive link to PTSD: Prewar trauma history (cumulative index of threatening life experiences); witnessing of atrocities or abusive violence considered deviant in the war zone (e.g., mutilation, killing civilians); perceived threat in the war zone (subjective assessment of fear); and stressful life events postwar. The following had a negative relationship to PTSD: Hardiness (e.g., sense of control, commitment to self, viewing change as a challenge) and functional social support postwar (perceived emotional sustenance and instrumental assistance from others).

Together, these six variables accounted for 72% of the variance in PTSD. For males, the same six variables emerged as predictive of PTSD, in addition to: age of arrival in Vietnam and structural social support post war (e.g., size and complexity of social network), which were negatively related to PTSD; and day-to-day discomforts in the war zone, which had a positive relationship to PTSD. These nine variables accounted for 70% of the total variance in males, indicating that very specific wartime experiences were important in the development of PTSD in soldiers.

One other feature not captured by these data is the fact that soldiers do not really have any control over whether they are exposed to these experiences. Draftees have little control over their induction into military service and during wartime have no effective control over who will be assigned combat duty and where. In contrast, exposure to the traumatic events of civilian life that would cause PTSD (e.g., significant life events) is far more controllable. Breslau, Davis, Andreski, and Peterson (1991) showed that exposure to traumatic events was significantly predicted by family history of psychiatric illness. This suggests that PTSD is mediated by two quite different mechanisms in general population versus military samples. Unlike military personnel, individuals in the general population are free to act on genetic predispositions to seek out or put themselves into situations where they are more likely to experience trauma—a form of gene-environment correlation—as opposed to military personnel, whose combat duty and environments are effectively preordained. Thus, any interplay with an underlying genetic liability in this sample may be the result of gene-environment interaction.

Do the Anxiety Disorders Share a Common Aetiological Heritage?

A final question concerns the nature of the relationship between the different anxiety disorder diagnoses. Clinically, these disorders are frequently comorbid with each other, which suggests that they share a common genetic basis. Early support for this hypothesis came from a study by Andrews et al. (1990), who examined twin concordance rates from 446 adult Australian twins who met *DSM-III* (1980) criteria for depression, dysthymia, OCD, social phobia, panic disorder or agoraphobia, and GAD. They found that if twins were concordant for one disorder, they were simultaneously concordant for others.

More recently, Kendler, Walters, Truett, et al. (1995) used multivariate genetic analyses to demonstrate that lifetime history of *DSM-III-R* (1987) phobia, GAD, panic, bulimia, major depression, and alcoholism shared a common genetic and environmental basis. An independent pathways model specifying two additive genetic factors, one shared and one nonshared environmental factor, provided a satisfactory explanation for their covariance. The two genetic factors appeared to delineate two broad domains of anxiety disorder. The first genetic factor accounted for the largest proportion of heritable influence on phobia (33%), panic disorder (32%), and bulimia (29%), and in total accounted for less than 7% of the variance on the remaining disorders. The second genetic factor was found to influence only GAD and major depression, accounting for 22% and 41% of the variance. This factor only accounted for 12% or less of the variance in the remaining four disorders. Alcoholism was minimally influenced by either genetic factor. Together, the common factors were found to account for only 7% of the variance on alcoholism, with 45% of the total variance attributable to alcohol-specific genetic factors.

The shared environmental (c^2) factor accounted for 41% of the total variance across all disorders, with the exception of bulimia, in which it accounted for approximately 2%. The single common nonshared environmental factor had the largest influence on GAD (38%) and depression (34%). Most of the nonshared environmental effects were found to be unique to each disorder, accounting for 29% to 49% of the total variance. These results clearly indicate that what we think of as a genetically homogenous set of disorders is actually quite an aetiologically diverse collection of conditions. The results also question whether some diagnoses such as GAD should continue to exist. As shown in this study and that of Kendler et al. (1992c), cited earlier, GAD appears to have more in common with major depression than any of the other anxiety disorders.

GENETIC EFFECTS ON PRECURSOR BEHAVIOR

Clinical research has shown that shyness is predictive of social phobia and that anxiety sensitivity is predictive of panic attacks. These relationships suggest that the anxiety disorders exist on a continuum of liability and represent an extreme form of normal behavior. As demonstrated in chapters 4 and 5, one way to test for this is to demonstrate that the relationship between normal and abnormal behavior has a common aetiological basis. The next section reviews this small but growing body of research on the anxiety disorders.

Precursors to Panic: Anxiety Sensitivity

A recognized risk factor for panic disorder is anxiety sensitivity (AS). AS is the fear of anxiety-related sensations arising from the belief that these sensations have harmful consequences (see Taylor, 1995). For example, an individual may fear that the sensation of heart palpitations is indicative of a serious, life-threatening condition such as a heart attack. According to expectancy theory, such an individual may become anxious whenever this symptom is experienced, and may tend to avoid activities or places that are felt to precipitate it. AS theory proposes that the higher an individual's level of AS, the more that individual is likely to experience anxiety symptoms as alarming, dangerous, and threatening. A biological basis for AS was hypothesized when Perna, Cocchi, and Bertani (1995) found that first-degree relatives of patients with panic disorder were more likely than first-degree relatives of controls to experience panic attacks during 35% CO_2 inhalation tests. They also found that panic disorder patients who panic in response to 35% CO_2 inhalation are more likely to have a positive family history of panic disorder than patients who are 35% CO_2-nonresponsive (Perna, Bertani, Caldirola, & Bellodi, 1996).

Stein, Jang, and Livesley (1999) showed that AS was indeed heritable. A sample of 179 MZ and 158 DZ general population twin pairs completed the Anxiety Sensitivity Index (ASI; Peterson & Reiss, 1992). The heritability of the total ASI score was 45%. The next task was to test whether the same genetic mechanisms influence normal- and extreme-range ASI scores. This test required that the heritability of extreme scores (group heritability or h_g^2), defined by a clinically significant threshold, be estimated and compared to the magnitude of genetic influences (indexed by h^2) on the entire range of scores (DeFries & Fulker, 1985, 1988; Plomin et al., 1991). Recall from chapter 3 that $h_g^2 = h^2$ is consistent with the hypothesis that normal- and extreme-range scores are influenced by the same genetic influences. This hypothesis is not supported if $h^2_g \neq h^2$. The clinical threshold for panic disorder on the ASI is a score of 25. Estimates of h^2_g for this score, as well as scores of 26 to 28, were also made to determine if even more extreme levels of AS were influenced by different genetic and environmental factors. The estimates of h^2_g for these thresholds ranged from 45% (ASI = 25) to 62% (ASI = 28). At first glance, the increased heritability associated with the most extreme ASI score suggests that additional genetic factors come into play to push AS over the threshold into panic disorder. However, the 45% to 62% estimates fall largely within the 95% confidence interval surrounding the 45% estimate (33%–59%), suggesting that high ASI scores are characteristic of panic disorder and those in the sub-clinical range are influenced by the same genetic factors.

A separate set of analyses factored the ASI items to estimate the heritability of different manifestations of AS. Three factors were extracted. The first was "physical concerns," the fear of physical symptoms due to the belief that arousal-related bodily sensations are indicative of physical illness. The second was "psychological concerns," or the fear of cognitive dyscontrol due to the belief that sensations like depersonalization are signs of mental illness. The third was "social concerns," the fear of publicly observable arousal-related experiences due to the belief that displays of anxiety will lead to public ridicule, embarrassment, and social censure. Heritability analyses revealed that the factors were differentially heritable. The psychological concerns factor was not heritable at all ($h^2_A = 0.0\%$, $c^2 = 11\%$, $e^2 = 89\%$), whereas the physical ($h^2_A = 35\%$, $c^2 = 0.0\%$, $e^2 = 65\%$) and social concerns ($h^2_A = 22\%$, $c^2 = 0.0\%$, $e^2 = 78\%$) factors were.

Despite any heritable basis, it is clear from these analyses that nonshared environmental factors account for the greatest proportion of the variance on ASI scores. The clinical literature suggests that one important class of events is childhood sexual or physical abuse (Stein et al., 1996). This experience could produce feelings of loss of bodily autonomy and concerns related to physiologic hyperarousal. Suffocation experiences (e.g., Bouwer & Stein, 1997) and other adverse respiratory experiences in childhood such as asthma (e.g., Smoller, Pollack, Otto, Rosenbau, & Kradin, 1996) might sensitize an individual to fear sensations associated with breathlessness. Learning to catastrophize about the occurrence of general bodily symptoms is thought to lead to higher than normal levels of AS.

Clinical research shows that the presentation of panic disorder is similar across genders (Oei, Wanstall, & Evans, 1990), but that the disorder is diagnosed more than twice as often in women (Kessler, McGonagle, & Zhao, 1994). There is some evidence that pharmacotherapies (e.g., alprazolam) yield better outcomes for females (e.g., Mavissakalian, 1985), although other reports have found no gender differences (Maier & Buller, 1988). Gender differences in the effectiveness of cognitive-behavioral therapies are also mixed. Hafner (1983) showed that men and women treated with *in vivo* exposure tended to be similar in terms of symptom severity and had approximately equal reductions in panic over the course of therapy, but others have not found this effect (e.g., Chambless & Gracely, 1988). Females have been consistently shown to score higher than males on physical concerns, whereas males score higher on the psychological and social concerns factors on the ASI (Stewart, Taylor, & Baker, 1990).

These reports suggest the intriguing possibility that gender differences in panic disorder may be due to gender differences in AS. Jang, Stein, Taylor, and Livesley (1999) investigated whether these gender differences were due to gender-specific genetic and environmental influences. The first step was to separately estimate the heritability of the ASI factors by gender. Among females, h^2_A was 48%, 33%, 37%, and 49% for physical, psychological, social concerns, and total ASI score, respectively, with the remainder accounted for by e^2 effects. In contrast, among males h^2_A was zero for all of these measures! Instead, significant c^2 effects were found, accounting for 42%, 46%, 36%, and 49% of the total variance, respectively. The finding that c^2 effects were so high among men as opposed to women is consistent with research by Watt, Stewart, and Cox (1998) indicating that social-learning factors such as early experiences that teach children to become fearful of anxiety-related sensations (e.g., by observing parents becoming alarmed about palpitations, shortness of breath, or trembling), play a greater role in shaping AS in men than in women.

Precursors to PTSD

Traumatic experiences and our responses to them are not limited to war zones. Any form of assault, natural disaster, car accident, or negative significant life event can also trigger symptoms of PTSD. A dimensional model would predict that these experiences and our responses to them are equivalent to those experienced by combat veterans. Stein, Jang, and Livesley (2002) set out to investigate this question by surveying 406 volunteer urban general population twin pairs recruited from Canada (222 MZ twin pairs and 184 DZ pairs) on lifetime exposure to traumatic events and their characteristic response to them. Twins were asked to report on their experience of several classes of traumatic events that ranged from car accidents and natural disasters to the death of a close family member or friend. Because it was a Canadian sample, virtually no twin had been in combat, but 75.4% of the total sample of individuals had experienced one or more of the other events. The list of traumatic events was factored and two factors describing traumatic events typically experienced by general population samples were extracted. The first factor described "assaultive events" (robbery, captivity, beating, sexual assault, other life threat) and the second was "nonassaultive events" (sudden family death, motor vehicle accident, fire, tornado, flood, or earthquake).

Two heritability analyses of assaultive and nonassaultive events were conducted. The first estimated the heritable basis of liability of exposure to assaultive trauma using data from all subjects, that is, whether or not they reported having experienced any trauma. Additive genetic effects accounted for 20.3%, $c^2 = 21.3\%$ and $e^2 = 58.4\%$. In contrast, a purely environmental model provided the best explanation of liability of exposure to nonassaultive trauma: $c^2 = 38.6\%$ and $e^2 = 61.5\%$. Moreover, the values of r_C and r_E between the types of exposure were estimated at .31 and −.20, suggesting that the environmental influences on assaultive and nonassaultive trauma are largely unrelated.

The second analysis estimated the heritable basis of PTSD symptoms conditional on actual trauma exposure by using data from pairs in which both members reported experiencing a traumatic event. Those who had reported an experience were asked to answer a set of questions in reference to the event that most disturbed them to assess DSM-IV (1994) PTSD cluster B through D symptoms. In this subsample of affected twins, additive genetic and nonshared environmental influences best explained the variance in assaultive trauma factor scores, and a purely environmental model provided the best explanation for the variance in nonassaultive trauma.

Heritability estimates for the symptoms were: reexperiencing (36%), avoidance (28%), numbing (36%), hyperarousal (29%), and total symptoms (38%). Nonshared effects accounted for the remaining variance. The r_g and r_e between liability to assaultive trauma exposure and PTSD symptoms were also computed. The values ranged from 0.71 to 0.83, suggesting that PTSD symptoms and the experience of trauma are inextricably linked by a common set of genetic factors. It is interesting to note that these estimates for PTSD symptoms and exposure to traumatic events come remarkably close to those derived from an exclusively male sample of combat veterans from the Vietnam Era Twin Registry. This finding is consistent with the hypothesis that the aetiological factors underlying PTSD symptoms in the general population are the same as those in combat veterans.

The finding that individuals' exposure to specific events is mediated by their genetic makeup is not a novel conclusion. Earlier, Kendler, Neale, Kessler, Heath, and Eaves (1993) showed that certain kinds of life events have a genetic basis. A sample of 2,315 twin pairs was surveyed on two kinds of life events experienced in the past year. The first was "network events," or events that had a primary impact on individuals in the respondent's social network (e.g., a death, illness or injury to member of the network, etc.). The second was "personal events," or events that had a primary impact on the respondent. Heritability analyses showed that network events were not heritable. Shared environmental effects were found to account for 32% to 45%, with nonshared environmental effect accounting for the remainder. In contrast, the personal events items were heritable. The heritability of experiencing marital difficulties was 14%; being robbed or assaulted = 33%; interpersonal difficulties = 39%; having financial problems = 18% with c^2 = 21%; illness or injury = 21%; and having problems at work = 18% with c^2 = 21%.

These studies show that certain kinds of events are partially under genetic control, but it is unlikely that the events themselves are heritable. Rather, what is more likely to be inherited are factors that influence the individual's risk for placing themselves in, or creating, potentially hazardous situations. Personality traits such as neuroticism have been implicated in this role (e.g., Fauerbach, Lawrence, & Schmidt, 2000) and other traits, such as sensation seeking, have been associated with increased risk for being a victim of rape (Kilpatrick, Resnick, Saunders, & Best,

1998). Koenen et al. (2002) reported that, among males, preexisting conduct disorder (which might be considered an early manifestation of antisocial personality traits) was a risk factor for both trauma exposure and subsequent PTSD symptoms using data from the Vietnam Era Twin Registry.

Following this up a bit further, Jang, Stein, Taylor, Asmundson, and Livesley (2003) examined the relationship between a wide range of normal and abnormal personality traits and exposure to assaultative and nonassaultive trauma. Normal personality was assessed using measures of the Big Five (FFI: Costa & McCrae, 1992) and "Gigantic Three" (EPQ-R Adult: Eysenck & Eysenck, 1992) personality domains. Personality dysfunction was assessed with 69 highly specific traits delineating personality disorder (DAPP: Livesley & Jackson, in press). Multiple regression analysis identified that traits describing antisocial personality characteristics were most predictive of assaultive trauma (see Fig. 6.1).

Precursors to Social Phobia

An extensive literature exists examining what is thought to be the subclinical form of social phobia—the fear of negative evaluation (FNE). Individuals with high FNE are sensitive to disapproval or criticism and are thus highly motivated to make a good impression on others (Leary & Kowalski, 1995). Cognitive models of social phobia posit that high FNE leads people with social phobia to believe that

		Predictors	h^2_A	r_G	r_E
1. Assaultive					
	DAPP	Juvenile antisocial behavior	.26*	.22*	.02
	DAPP	Self-damaging acts	.26*	.24*	.10
	FFI	Openness	.22*	.14*	.03
	DAPP	Lack of empathy	.19*	-.07	.00
	DAPP	Restricted expression of affect	.13*	-.06	.00
	DPQ-R	Psychoticism	.10*	.36*	.06
$R^2_{Adjusted} = .24$					
2. Non-assaultive					
	DAPP	Conscientiousness	-.17*		
	DAPP	Impulsivity	.15*		
	DAPP	Inhibited sexuality	-.13*		
	DAPP	Desire for improved affiliative relationships	.16*		
	EPQ-R	Neuroticism	-.12*		
$R^2_{Adjusted} = .06$					

FIG. 6.1. Personality predictors of assaultive and nonassaultive trauma exposure. *$p < .05$.

they are in danger when exposed to possible scrutiny by others, and that rejection or loss of status is likely to result (Stopa & Clark, 2000). These beliefs are thought to lead to avoidance patterns that subsequently reinforce these convictions (e.g., Rapee & Heimberg, 1997).

Studies have shown that social phobia runs in families (e.g., Mannuzza et al., 1995; Stein, Chartier, Kozak, Hazenetal, et al., 1998). Rates of social phobia and scores on measures of FNE are higher in families of probands with social phobia (Stein, Chartier, Kozak, & Jang, 2001). Of particular interest are the results of the family- and community-based research suggesting that social phobia is part of a continuum bounded by mild (i.e., normative) shyness at one end and avoidant personality disorder at the other (Stein & Chavira, 1998; Tillfors et al., 2001; van Velsen, Emmelkamp, & Scholing, 2000). Stein, Jang, and Livesley (2002) examined this issue with a multivariate genetic analysis of FNE and traits delineating avoidant personality disorder in a sample of 437 pairs of general population twins. The twins completed a brief version of the Fear of Negative Evaluation Scale (BFNE: Watson & Friend, 1969) and the DAPP. The first set of analyses established that the BFNE was heritable ($h^2_B = 48\%$). The next set of analyses showed that the genetic influences underlying traits delineating avoidant personality disorder overlapped substantially with the genetic influences on FNE: The genetic correlations between BFNE scores and DAPP submissiveness, anxiousness, and social avoidance ranged from 0.78 to 0.80.

The results show that a cognitive dimension central to the phenomenology and aetiology of social phobia is heritable and that many of the same genes that influence FNE appear to influence a cluster of anxiety-related personality characteristics. These results have several implications. First, they suggest that a common set of genes influence vulnerability to these Axis I and Axis II disorders and, if replicated, would support the growing consensus that social phobia on Axis I and avoidant personality disorder on Axis II are really classifications of the same construct. This would provide support for the argument that the division of Axis I and II disorders, although heuristically convenient, is often not empirically supported (e.g., Widiger, 2003). The findings may also be informative regarding the composition of particular Axis II diagnostic criteria. One of the defining criteria of *DSM-IV* (1994) avoidant personality disorder—intimacy problems—had a negligible genetic correlation with FNE. This suggests that there may be heterogeneity within the avoidant personality disorder diagnostic category, with presence of intimacy problems delineating a form of the disorder that is aetiologically distinct from the social-anxiety-related form. This hypothesis deserves to be tested in future family and twin studies.

MODELS OF ACQUISITION

The first two sections of this chapter reviewed the magnitude of genetic and environmental effects and it was shown that heritable influences were consistently modest (e.g., accounting for less than 50% of the total variability) across the anxiety disorder diagnoses and their premorbid forms. More interestingly, the research also detected the presence of c^2 effects, further highlighting the role of the environment, experience, and learning on these disorders. However, the fact that genetic influences are even present ($h^2 \neq 0$) is inconsistent with a strict learning model, suggesting that the anxiety disorders are a product of the interplay of genetic and environmental effects. This last section of the chapter presents recent work that integrates the elements of learning and genetics and explores how they converge to produce disorder.

How do learning and experience combine with genetic liabilities to produce disorder? A popular hypothesis is the classical diathesis-stress model, which predicts that an inverse relationship exists between the level of diathesis (genetic liability) and the level of onset-related environmental trauma. Affected individuals whose onset was associated with high levels of trauma should, on average, have lower levels of disease liability than affected individuals with little or no trauma associated with onset.

Kendler, Meyers, and Prescott (2002) conducted a study that directly tested the classical diathesis-stress model as it applies to the development of phobias and other irrational fears. The study utilized the five models of phobia acquisition from social learning theory. The first is that fear develops as a result of traumatic events; the second is that fear develops as a consequence of observing traumatic events happening to others; the third is that fear develops from the observation of fear or avoidance behaviors in others; the fourth is that subjects are taught to be afraid; and the fifth is that they have no memory of how or why the fear developed (e.g., commonly indicated by the response of phobic patients, "I've just always been afraid of that").

These models imply different levels of genetic liability. It was hypothesized that those with no memory of a traumatic event (Model 5) would tend to have the highest levels of genetic liability. "Not remembering" is associated with the highest genetic risk because the onset of fear is "spontaneous" and is not associated by learning or observation with any traumatic event. At the other end of the spectrum, people who report that the onset of fear was associated with a major trauma (Model 1) should have low to average genetic liability. This model is considered the least genetic because the person can identify a specific event where they learned to be fearful. As such, it predicts that among phobics there is an inverse relationship between the level of genetic liability and the level of environmental trauma (see Fig. 6.2).

Contrary to their prediction, Kendler et al. (2002) found that the risk of phobia was significantly lower in cotwins who reported no memory of how they acquired their phobia (those at greatest genetic risk), versus those who recalled a specific event (those at the lowest genetic risk) suggesting that genetic liability to phobia does not have much influence on their acquisition. Kendler and colleagues concluded that their test of the diathesis-stress model for phobias failed. One explanation offered for the failure of the diathesis-stress model is that this version of it simply does not apply to phobias.

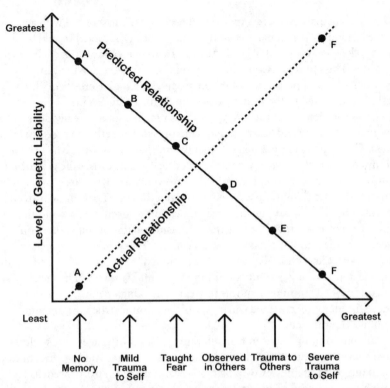

FIG. 6.2.   Level of environmental trauma associated with fear acquisition. Adapted from "The Etiology of Phobias: An Evaluation of the Stress-Diathesis Model," by K. S. Kendler, J. Myers, and C. A. Prescott, 2002, *Archives of General Psychiatry, 59*, p. 244. Copyright 2002 by American Medical Association. Adapted with permission.

The diathesis-stress model illustrated in Figure 6.2 it is very much a "one stress— one illness model". The type of stress and the magnitude of stress experienced by an individual that has inherited a particular genetic liability will have a direct effect in the development of a particular kind of behavior. It also suggests each kind and/or magnitude of stressful event is keyed to largely specific behavioral responses. However, the multivariate genetic analyses of the anxiety disorders reviewed earlier suggest that this kind of one stress-one illness model is too simple. For example, the phobias have been shown to be comorbid with many other disorders and that some of that comorbidity is attributable to genetic and environmental influences in common. As such, stressors that affect the other disorders (for the sake of this hypothetical example, depression) will also have an indirect effect on the phobias. If the multivariate genetic models are correct, a depressogenic event can influence phobia but under a classical diathesis-stress model, depressogenic stressors can be overlooked as risk factor for phobia because they are understood as being important only in depression. The expectation of the classical diathesis-stress model that each stress is associated with a particular stress response is a bit narrow. Rather, the scope of the model should be broadened to take into account that each stressor can invoke a wide variety of behavioral responses. This approach would be consistent with the research in health psychology, where the best predictors of mood are the summative effects of "life's daily hassles" as opposed to the influence of a single major life event.

Another limitation of the diathesis-stress model is that it really does not say how genetic liability and environmental factors work together to produce mental illness. The graph in Fig. 6.2 suggests that the mechanism is some kind of gene-environment interaction where exposure to critical events causes the genetic liability for irrational fear to come online. However, recent research by Hettema, Annas, and Neale (2003) suggests that this is not the case. They found instead that genetics influence the rate at which fear conditioning occurs. Fear conditioning is a basic form of associative learning that is considered important in the acquisition of fears, phobias, and possibly anxiety in general. Fear conditioning occurs when fear is associated with a neutral (or "conditioned") stimulus after being paired with a fear-provoking (or "unconditioned stimulus") such as an electric shock. The conditioned stimulus acquires the fear provoking response of the unconditioned stimulus after repeated pairings, which continues when the unconditioned stimulus is eliminated.

Fear conditioning between fear-relevant (pictures of snakes and spiders) and fear-irrelevant (pictures of circles and triangles) stimuli and mild electric shock was carried out on 173 same-sex twin pairs (90 MZ and 83 DZ) from Sweden. The fear response was assessed using electrodermal skin conduction. Heritability analysis showed that the fear-conditioning process was moderately heritable, accounting for 35% to 45% of the variability in electrodermal skin conduction. More interestingly, multivariate genetic models showed that two genetic factors underlie fear conditioning. The first genetic factor appears to influence the unlearning of fear, that is, the nonassociative processes of habituation to the conditioned stimulus. The second genetic factor appears to influence the acquisition of fear. Their analyses also showed that the relevance of the fear stimuli appears to be differentially heritable. The heritability of the fear response to spiders and snakes was generally higher than the fear response to geometric shapes. This is consistent with evolutionary theories that humans are primed to automatically and selectively attend to specific stimuli that are important for survival. They also noted that, clinically, the fear response to fear-relevant stimuli like spiders and snakes is harder to extinguish than fear-irrelevant stimuli.

SUMMARY

Of all the major psychopathologies, the anxiety disorders are influenced most by nonheritable factors. Heritability of OCD, panic disorder, GAD, PTSD, and the phobias typically falls in the 30% range, with shared and nonshared environmental influences accounting for the remainder. Similar estimates have been reported for premorbid forms of these disorders. Heritability estimates of FNE are similar to those of social phobia. These findings are supportive of a dimensional model of anxiety disorders.

In the clinical and research literature, models of learning have figured prominently. Learning-based psychotherapies, including cognitive-behavioral therapy, have been shown to be the most successful treatments for these disorders. This fact, coupled with the size of the environmental effect, has given rise to the suggestion that the learning process is an important source of c^2 and e^2 effects. This idea was investigated by testing how phobias are acquired. Studies have shown that phobias are not acquired by simple exposure to different kinds of threatening events. Rather, genetic factors were found to play a key role in moderating the effect of these exposures by influencing the rate by which fear associations are acquired or extinguished.

Chapter 7

Substance Use Problems

There is little doubt that substance use runs in families, as demonstrated by Merikangas and Avenevoli (2000) in an 8-year longitudinal family study of 340 substance use probands, 1,626 first-degree relatives and a sample of community-based controls. They found significant rates of family aggregation for alcohol abuse (odds ratio = 3.5, 95% CI = 1.3–9.4), dependence (OR = 3.1, 95% CI = 1.1–9.1), and alcohol use (OR = 1.8, 95% CI = 1.0–3.2), as well as cannabis use (OR = 2.7, 95% CI = 1.4–5.0), abuse (OR = 2.9, 95% CI = .09–9.8), and dependence (OR = 3.2, 95% CI = 1.2–8.6). With drugs other than cannabis, a significant familial aggregation was also found (OR = 3.3, 95% CI = 1.3–8.3) with a marked difference in rates of dependence (OR = 0.8, 95% CI = .10–8.8) versus abuse (OR = 1.6, 95% CI = 0.2–11.4).

The familial basis of substance use problems highlights the importance of family-based prevention programs. In particular, Merikangas and Avenevoli (2000) noted that targeted prevention should be geared toward offspring of substance abusers, even those who have not been identified in treatment settings. Second, because only a minority of those who experiment with drugs proceed to harmful use, public health prevention efforts would be more effective if targeted at those who are most likely to continue to abuse drugs and suffer a personal and social impact. Finally, their results highlight the importance of delaying or preventing transition from use to harmful use and preventing dependence rather than experimentation.

The remainder of this chapter examines these results in a little detail; in particular the behavioral genetic research on the relationship between substances, the progression from use to dependence, and the relationship between substance use and other psychopathology. The chapter is divided into three broad sections. The first reviews molecular univariate and multivariate genetic research on alcohol, tobacco, and illicit drug use. The second evaluates the evidence for the hypothesized "addictive personality" and also reviews the relationship between substance use and other psychopathology. The third reviews the environmental factors that increase the risk for substance use, and those that protect against it.

ALCOHOL

The Heritability of Male Alcoholism

Among males, however alcoholism is defined, the heritability estimates consistently fall in the 45% to 50% range. Prescott and Kendler (1999) estimated the heritability (h^2_A) of male twins who met the criteria for DSM-III-R (1987) alcohol dependence at 49% (95% CI: 39%–58%), with the remaining 51% (42%–61%) due to e^2 effects. When the newer DSM-IV (1994) dependence criteria were applied, the estimates remained stable: $h^2_A = 51\%$ (95% CI: 41%–60%) and $e^2 = 49\%$ (95% CI: 40%–59%). The heritability of DSM-III-R alcohol abuse was $h^2_A = 55\%$ (95% CI: 46%–63%) and $e^2 = 45\%$ (95% CI: 37%–54%). Application of the newer DSM-IV criteria did not change the estimate: $h^2_A = 58\%$ (50%–66%) and $e^2 = 42\%$ (34%–52%). When all twins suffering from abuse or dependence were pooled, the estimates remained similar: $h^2_A = 55\%$ (95% CI: 47%–63%) and $e^2 = 45\%$ (95% CI: 37%–53%), and using DSM-III-R criteria, h^2_A was estimated at 56% (95% CI: 48%–64%) and $e^2 = 44\%$ (95% CI: 36%–52%).

Prescott and Kendler (1999) next pooled unaffected pairs, pairs suffering from abuse, and pairs suffering from dependence in a single analysis. The heritability of DSM-III-R (1987) criteria was $h^2_A = 48\%$ (41%–56%), with $e^2 = 52\%$ (44%–59%); by DSM-IV (1994) criteria $h^2_A = 56\%$ (49%–64%), with $e^2 = 44\%$ (36%–51%). The findings are consistent with the idea that alcohol problems exist on a continuum of liability (e.g., Heath, Bucholz, & Slutske, 1994), because the heritability estimate did not change across groups of male twins with differing levels of alcohol problems. This study is also notable because no shared family effects were found for lifetime abuse and dependence. This finding runs counter to popular theories that alcohol problems are the result of social class or parental disciplinary practices (assuming that parents applied them equally to all children in the family) and drinking behaviors (e.g., Holmes & Robins, 1988).

Although shared environmental effects did not appear to play a role in the development of alcohol use problems, they have been shown to play a significant role in treatment seeking. Prescott and Kendler (1996) identified a sample of twins who met the diagnostic criteria for abuse or dependence and had either voluntarily reported for treatment in an alcohol or substance use program or had been court-ordered into an outpatient program following an alcohol-related offense. A total of 108 MZ and 109 DZ pairs were identified, and heritability analysis estimated DSM-IV (1994): alcohol dependence at $h^2_A = 63\%$, $c^2 = 17\%$, $e^2 = 20\%$; for DSM-IV alcohol abuse $h^2_A = 48\%$, $c^2 = 34\%$, $e^2 = 18\%$; and for DSM-IV abuse or dependence combined: $h^2_A = 48\%$, $c^2 = 37\%$, $e^2 = 15\%$.

They found similar results using a sample of Swedish males who were registered with the Swedish Temperance Board, whose mandate is to follow up individuals who were seen in legal or medical settings with problems of alcohol abuse. Note that alcohol abuse is not diagnosed in the *DSM-III-R* (1987) or other medical sense, but rather in a legal sense. Males were registered if they had engaged in: (a) drunkenness, (b) illegal manufacture or sale of alcohol (not included in the analyses), (c) driving under the influence of alcohol, or (d) committing a crime while drinking. In a sample of 1,258 twin pairs (born between 1902 and 1949) registered with this board, the heritability of this broad definition alcoholism was $h^2_A = 54\%$, $c^2 = 14\%$ (95% CI: 8%–19%), and $e^2 = 32\%$.

Heritability of Female Alcoholism

Heritability of alcohol abuse in women mirrors that in men. In a sample of 1,030 pairs of female twins, the heritability of *DSM-III-R* (1987) alcoholism with dependence tolerance was 50%; alcoholism with or without dependence tolerance was 56%, and alcoholism with or without dependence or problem drinking was 61% (Kendler, Heath, Neale, Kessler, & Eaves, 1992). Nonshared environmental effects (e^2) accounted for the remainder. When all three definitions were pooled, $h^2_A = 58\%$ and $e^2 = 42\%$. Similar estimates were obtained in Australia (Heath et al., 1997). This sample consisted of 1,706 MZ female pairs, 901 MZ male pairs, 1,113 DZ female pairs, 630 DZ male pairs, and 1,617 DZ opposite-sex pairs drawn from the general population (who, consequently, are likely suffer from less severe forms of alcohol use problems). Heritability analysis estimated the additive genetic effects (h^2_A) of *DSM-III-R* alcoholism in both females and males at 64% (95% CI: 32%–73%) with nonshared environmental effects accounting for the remaining 35% (27%–47%).

However, McGue, Pickens, and Svikis (1992) did not find such consistent results across gender. In 404 twin pairs recruited from an alcohol abuse treatment center (MZ male = 85, DZ male = 96, MZ female = 44, DZ female = 43, DZ opposite-sex = 88) who were diagnosed with *DSM-III* (1980) criteria for alcohol abuse or dependence, male $h^2_A = 56\%$ ($\pm$ 17.5%), $c^2 = 33\%$ ($\pm$ 12.5%), and $e^2 = 12.6\%$ ($\pm$ 3.4%). In stark contrast, female heritability was 0.0%, $c^2 = 63\%$ ($\pm$ 4.9%), and $e^2 = 37\%$ ($\pm$ 4.9). These results suggest that quite different genetic and environmental effects may be involved in male and female alcoholism. Of particular interest are the significant c^2 effects that appear to be characteristic of samples recruited from treatment settings.

To resolve this issue, Prescott, Aggen, and Kendler (2000) tested whether males and females were directly affected by gender-specific genetic and environmental influences. They surveyed 5,091 male and 4,168 female twins clinically chosen from the general population on *DSM-IV* (1994) alcohol abuse and dependence criteria. For same-sex female twin pairs, alcohol dependence was $h^2_A = 59\%$ (95% CI: 45%–72%); for abuse or dependence, $h^2_A = 66\%$ (95% CI: 54%–76%); and for all definitions combined, $h^2_A = 59\%$ (95% CI: 44%–71%). For males, alcohol dependence was $h^2_A = 52\%$ (95% CI: 42%–58%); for abuse or dependence, $h^2_A = 56\%$ (95% CI: 48% –64%); and for all definitions combined $h^2_A = 53\%$ (95% CI: 46%–60%).

Once the heritability of male and female alcoholism had been established, they tested whether the genetic factors influencing males were the same as those influencing females. This was accomplished by estimating the genetic correlation (r_G) between the same-sex and opposite-sex twin pairs. For alcohol dependence, r_G was a modest .24 (95% CI: .04–.45). When the definition was expanded to include abuse or dependence, $r_G = .22$ (95% CI: .06–.38). For all diagnoses combined, r_G remained a modest .22 (95% CI: .07–.38), suggesting that each gender is influenced largely by gender-specific genetic factors.

Heritability by Age

The discussion so far has concentrated on point estimates—the heritability of definitions of alcohol problems at a specific point in time. Does it seem reasonable to assume that the same type and magnitude of genetic and environmental factors are important in the development of alcohol problems across the lifespan? Moreover, it is possible that some of the gender-specific variability is related to age.

McGue et al. (1992) found that genetic factors in males played a critical role at the age of onset of *DSM-III* (1980) alcohol abuse or dependence compared to other points in the lifespan. Age of onset was defined by the proband's age at first symptom. Early onset was defined by first symptom at age 20 or younger, and late onset by appearance of first symptom at age 21 or older. In the early-onset group, the h^2_A for males = 72.5% (± 17.5%) and for females = 0%. Shared environmental factors (c^2) were 23.2% (± 17.4%) in males and 73.2% (± 6.1%) in females, with e^2 = 4.3% (± 2.2%) in males and 26.8% (± 6.1%) in females. However, in the late-onset group, h^2_A for males dropped to 29.5% (± 26.4%), $c^2 = 37.2\%$ (± 20.3%), and $e^2 = 33.3\%$ (± 9.7%). For late-onset females, h^2_A remained at 0%, $c^2 = 52.5\%$ (± 7.6%), and $e^2 = 47.5\%$ (± 7.6%).

Prescott, Hewitt, Truett, and Heath's (1994) study of 3,049 female and 1,070 male twins age 50 to 96 showed that genetic influences on alcohol problems decrease with age. Across a nearly 50-year span, h^2_A ranged from 20% to 48%, c^2 effects ranged from 7% to 22%, and e^2 effects ranged from 36% to 59%. Such age-related genetic differences, coupled with epidemiologic research showing that early age of onset is associated with an increased risk of developing alcohol dependence or abuse (e.g., Grant & Dawson, 1997), has led some to suggest that preventing early alcohol use will decrease later rates of problem drinking. For example, Pedersen and Skrondal (1998) noted that "a 10% delay in debut age will lead to a 35% decrease in subsequent alcohol consumption" (p. 32). Such a statement would be supported if the relationship between age of onset and later diagnosis had a genetic basis. To test this, Prescott and Kendler (1999) first estimated the observed relationship between age of onset (first drink) and later dependence. They found that age of onset accounted for approximately 29% of the total variance in male and female *DSM-IV* (1994) alcohol dependence. For alcohol abuse, age of drinking onset accounted for 12% of variability in females and 3% in males. Genetic analyses showed that virtually all (95%–99%) of these observed relationships were directly attributable to genetic influences. However, the interpretation of these results must be tempered by the fact that the initial relationship between age of onset and later alcohol problems is modest, yielding lukewarm support for delaying age of first drink as a preventative technique for subsequent alcohol abuse and dependence.

Molecular Genetics of Alcoholism

There is a huge body of literature reporting the results of linkage and association studies of alcohol use and other substances. As with all the molecular genetic research surveyed so far, many reports have implicated specific genes in alcohol use, but just as many have suggested that the same genes are not influential. Rather than providing a comprehensive review of this literature for each substance, this section presents a few recent examples of alcohol studies to highlight some interesting trends in this research.

The dopamine system has been a focus of research because of some early associations between the dopamine D2 receptor locus and alcoholism (e.g., Blum et al., 1990). However, these results were not replicated (e.g., Bolos et al., 1990) and attention has shifted to other dopaminergic systems. The catechol-o-methyltransferase (COMT) enzyme has come under scrutiny because it plays a role in the metabolism of dopamine. Lachman et al. (1996) suggested that a polymorphism in the COMT gene results in a three- to four-fold difference in COMT enzyme activity that contributes to the aetiology of mental disorders such as bipolar disorder and alcoholism. Because ethanol-induced euphoria is associated with the rapid release of dopamine in limbic areas, it was considered conceivable that subjects who inherited the low-activity version of the COMT allele would have a relatively low dopamine-inactivation rate, and therefore would be more vulnerable to the development of ethanol dependence. Tiihonen et al. (1999) tested this hypothesis by genotyping a sample of late-onset alcoholics in Finland and found a significantly higher frequency of the low-activity allele.

Lusher, Ebersole, and Ball (2000) found a relationship between the dopamine D4 receptor (DRD4) gene and severity of dependence. The original purpose of the study was to replicate earlier reports that there was an excessive frequency of the long-long (LL) allele in the coding sequence of the DRD4 gene in opiate-dependent subjects. Data were collected on a sample of 60 opiate-dependent, 51 alcohol-dependent, and 64 normal, healthy control subjects and no significant association was found between the DRD4 polymorphism and opiate or alcohol abuse. However, a relationship between the LL allele and severity of alcohol and opiate dependence was found. The subjects who carried the LL form rated their severity of dependence significantly higher than those who had the short-short (SS) allele. Lush et al. concluded that the DRD4 gene does not directly influence vulnerability to substance dependence; rather, possession of the LL genotype significantly increased severity of dependence.

Another recent neurochemical of interest is the neuropeptide cholecystokinin (CCK) because one of its several functions is to modulate the release of dopamine in brain areas involved in reinforcement and reward behavior. Vanakoski, Virkkunen, Naukkarinen, and Goldman (2001) examined the association of CCK-system genes (CCK, CCK(A), and CCK(B) receptor genes) and alcohol dependence. Their sample was 257 alcohol-dependent probands assessed using *DSM-III-R* (1987) criteria from Finland, genotyped for three variants of the CCK-receptor polymorphisms. The allele frequencies were compared between 150 unrelated healthy Finnish controls and 107 unrelated alcohol-dependent subjects who were also criminal offenders. It was found that the frequency of the CCK polymorphisms were not significantly different between the groups.

Hesselbrock, Begleiter, Porjesz, O'Connor, and Bauer (2001) wrote that a problem with genotyping studies is that the clinical heterogeneity of the disorder results in a poorly defined phenotype for genetic analysis. They suggested that rather than relying on clinical definitions of alcoholism, better results may be obtained by switching to a diagnostic phenotype for alcoholism grounded in the examination of neurobiological correlates of the disorder. One endophenotype that has received much attention is the P300 event-related brain potentials (ERP) wave form. ERPs are recordings of neuroelectrical activity in response to stimuli recorded by electrodes on the scalp. Common stimuli include flashing lights, reactions to a short emotionally laden video clip, or noises. ERP has been shown to be a valid neurobiological correlate of alcoholism in both genders (Prabhu et al., 2001).

Using data from the Collaborative Study on the Genetics of Alcoholism (COGA), Hesselbrock et al. (2001) reported significant reductions in P300 amplitude between alcoholics and non-alcoholics; between unaffected relatives of alcoholics and relatives of controls; and between unaffected offspring of alcoholic fathers and offspring of controls. Almasy et al. (2001) conducted a genome-wide scan of P300 responses to a semantic priming task on 604 individuals in 100 pedigrees, ascertained as part of the COGA project. They showed that the P300 wave form was significantly heritable—in the 40%–50% range—and reported significant evidence of linkage to chromosome 5 and suggestive evidence of linkage to chromosome 4.

Heritability of Tobacco Use

Heath, Martin, Lynskey, Todorov, and Madden (2002) examined whether smoking initiation and persistence shared a common genetic and environmental basis. Initiation and persistence data were collected from 692 MZ female, 312 MZ male, 420 DZ female, 157 DZ male, and 427 DZ opposite-sex twin pairs. Smoking initiation was assessed using a scale containing items such as "never smoked" and "onset after 18 years of age." Persistence was simply assessed as either "still smoking" or "quit smoking." For initiation, h^2_B was 62.6% in females and only 21.7% in males. Shared environment (c^2) accounted for 10.5% in females and 41.5% in males. Quite a different result was found for persistence. In both genders, h^2_A was estimated at 42.2%; c^2 accounted for 8.7% in males and 10.4% in females, with nonshared effects (e^2) accounting for the remaining 49.2% of the variability in males and 47.4% in females. They also found that the genetic factors influencing initiation and persistence were largely unique to each domain. In females, r_G between initiation and persistence was 0.28, with $r_E = -.02$; among males, $r_G = 0.11$ and $r_E = -.39$.

Kendler, Neale, et al. (1999) reported similar results in a study of over 1,000 female twin pairs who answered questions on smoking initiation and nicotine dependence. Smoking initiation was assessed with questions such as, "Have you ever smoked regularly— at least seven cigarettes per week, for at least a month?" to identify a period when respondents smoked most heavily. Nicotine dependence was assessed using the eight-item Fagerstrom Tolerance Questionnaire (Fagerstrom & Schneider, 1989) and four *DSM-IV* (1994) drug dependence criteria. Factoring these variables yielded a single measure of dependence defined by the number of minutes before first cigarette after waking, number of cigarettes per day when smoking most heavily, checking to make sure cigarettes were available, difficulty refraining where forbidden, and strength of craving when denied.

Kendler, Neale, et al. (1999) fit a model that simultaneously estimated the additive genetic, shared environmental, and nonshared environmental effects for initiation and nicotine dependence, weighted by their relationship to each other (*b*). They found the heritability of smoking initiation at $h^2_A = 85\%$, $c^2 = 0.0$, and $e^2 = 15\%$. For nicotine dependence, $h^2_A = 22\%$, $c^2 = 0.0$, and $e^2 = 19\%$. The value of *b* was .77 and when squared showed that 59% of the total genetic and environment-based liabilities on smoking dependence are shared with smoking initiation.

Heritability of Caffeine Use

Recent behavioral genetic research on caffeine use has established that it is highly heritable and that heritability plays a role in the amount of caffeine consumed. Kendler and Prescott (1999b) estimated h^2_B on a sample of 486 MZ and 335 DZ female twin pairs for caffeine use at 40%, whereas heavy caffeine use (near-daily consumption of 625 mg or more per day) was 77%. They also estimated the heritability of caffeine toxicity by asking if the person felt ill, shaky, or jittery after drinking caffeinated beverages; tolerance was assessed using *DSM-III-R* (1987) criteria (e.g., if you drank the same amount, did it have less effect than before); and caffeine withdrawal was assessed using *DSM-IV* (1994) criteria (e.g., presence of headaches and one of the following: marked fatigue and drowsiness, marked anxiety or depression, or nausea and vomiting after trying to stop or cut down consumption). The heritability of toxicity (h^2_A) was 45% and 40% for tolerance. For withdrawal, the genetic effect was completely nonadditive, with h^2_d estimated at 35%. All of the remaining influence was attributable to e^2 effects. The differential heritability of caffeine use and its symptoms suggests that there are specific genetic factors that differentiate extreme use and its consequences.

The Heritability of Illicit Drug Use

There are a variety of psychoactive substances available and their use has become a focus of behavioral genetic research. As with alcohol, nicotine, and caffeine, the use of these drugs has been examined in the contexts of initiation, abuse, and dependence. One of the best examples is a study by Kendler, Karkowski, Corey, Prescott, and Neale (1999) that estimated the heritability of initiation and misuse of a number of psychoactive substances. A sample of 1,934 female twin pairs was interviewed for lifetime use of cannabis, sedatives, stimulants, cocaine, hallucinogens, inhalants, and over-the-counter (OTC) medications. Given the low endorsement rates of certain substances, they were grouped into three classes: (a) any kind of illicit drug use, (b) cannabis, and (c) stimulants (including amphetamines, methylphenidate, and methedrine, and cocaine and its derivatives).

Kendler, Karkowski, et al. (1999) estimated the heritability of initiation and misuse in each substance class, as well as the degree to which initiation and dependence shared a common genetic and environmental basis (b). For any kind of illicit drug use, $h^2_{initiation} = 49\%$, $c^2_{initiation} = 28\%$, and $e^2_{initiation} = 23\%$; and $h^2_{misuse} = 23\%$, $c^2_{misuse} = 0.0\%$, and $e^2_{misuse} = 24\%$, in which 53% of the genetic and environmental factors are common (b^2) to initiation and misuse. For cannabis, the results are similar: $h^2_{initiation} = 46\%$, $c^2_{initiation} = 29\%$, and $e^2_{initiation} = 25\%$; and $h^2_{misuse} = 17\%$, $c^2_{misuse} = 0.0\%$, and $e^2_{misuse} = 17\%$, in which 66% of the genetic and environmental factors are common (b^2) to cannabis initiation and misuse.

Stimulant use showed a different pattern. Initiation of stimulant use appeared to be entirely learned: $h^2_{initiation} = 0.0\%$, $c^2_{initiation} = 63\%$, and $e^2_{initiation} = 37\%$. However, stimulant misuse was moderately heritable: $h^2_{misuse} = 25\%$, $c^2_{misuse} = 0.0\%$, and $e^2_{misuse} = 4\%$, with 77% of the environmental effects common to initiation and subsequent abuse.

The most interesting aspect of this study is that c^2 effects were detected on all three classes of substance initiation. Kendler, Karkowski, et al. (1999) speculated that these environmental factors might include religious beliefs, attitudes toward drug use, parental monitoring during adolescence, parental use of licit substances such as nicotine and alcohol, common peer group pressures, and availability. They also suggested that the genetic factors underlying initiation might be the same as those underlying personality traits such as novelty seeking or extraversion—traits that influence a person's willingness to experiment. Once initiation had occurred, they explained that another set of genetic factors appeared to play a role in maintaining their use. This relationship is not unlike that between certain types of exposure to environmental toxins and the genetic risk for cancer. Such genes have no impact on the liability to cancer unless they encounter toxins.

Tsuang et al. (1998) showed that several different drug classes were also influenced by a common aetiology. Their sample consisted of 3,372 male twin pairs who were Vietnam veterans. The twins were assessed for abuse and dependence symptoms using *DSM-III-R* (1987) criteria and were interviewed on a wide variety of substances such as marijuana use (including hashish), stimulant use (including amphetamines, cocaine, and crack), sedatives (e.g., barbiturates, valium, Librium, tranquilizers, Xanax, and quaaludes), heroin and opiates (including codeine, Demerol, morphine, Percodan, methadone, and opium), and psychedelics (including lysergic acid diethylamide, mescaline, peyote, and psilocybin).

First, they found that abuse in any category was associated with a marked increase in the probability of abusing every other category of drugs. Second, the multivariate genetic analysis showed that heritability of marijuana, stimulant, sedative, opiate, and hallucinogen use due to the common genetic factor was estimated at 22%, 24%, 22%, 16%, and 26%, respectively. In contrast, unique genetic factors were generally much smaller and accounted for 11%, 9%, 5%, 38%, and 0.0% respectively. A significant proportion of the total nonshared environmental variance was also found to be common to the five categories, accounting for 38% of the total variance for marijuana use, 48% for stimulant use, 56% for sedatives, 33% for heroin, and 53% for psychedelic use.

The Causes of Comorbidity

The previous sections examined the heritable bases of different forms of substance use problems. This section reviews some of the literature determining whether all forms of substance use share a common aetiology. Han, McGue, and Iacono (1999) examined this question on a population-based sample of 327 MZ and 174 DZ adolescent twin pairs (ages 17-18) from Minnesota. They assessed tobacco use, lifetime alcohol use, and drug abuse on an "ever used versus never used" basis. Drug use included marijuana, stimulants, tranquilizers, quaaludes, cadrines, inhalants, nonprescription drugs, cocaine, psychedelics, and opiates. They began by estimating the heritability of substance use for each gender. Among males, the heritability (h^2_A) was 59% for tobacco use, 60% for alcohol use, and 33% for drug use. For females, heritabilities (h^2_A) were much lower at 11% for tobacco, 10% for alcohol, and 23% for drugs. Among males, shared environmental influences (c^2) accounted for 18%, 23%, and 23%; and c^2 was 71%, 68%, and 36% in females, respectively.

Multivariate genetic analyses showed that these substances did share a common aetiological basis. A single additive genetic factor accounted for 23% of the observed correlation among tobacco, alcohol, and drug use. A shared environmental factor accounted for 63% of the covariance among these substances. In contrast, a single nonshared environmental factor accounted for only 14% of the relationship among these substances. These findings suggest that genetic factors only modestly affect the risk for poly-substance use, but that factors within the home have the greatest influence on whether using one substance increases the risk for using others.

Jang, Livesley, and Vernon (1995) found similar results. Their analyses extracted three modestly overlapping genetic factors. The first genetic factor appeared to have the greatest impact on normal alcohol use. The second genetic factor influenced experimentation with illicit drug use. However, the third genetic factor influenced both alcohol and illicit drug use, specifically, "pathological" misuse of alcohol and drugs. The alcohol and drug use items defining this factor were "I drank so much that I could not remember what happened," "I drank so much I got into trouble," and "Drug use caused me to take time off work or school." In contrast, the shared and nonshared influences did not differentiate between type of substance or severity in the same way. The environmental effects were more generalized, influencing the variability of all substances and severity.

Similar patterns have been detected in family study designs. Bierut et al. (1998) compared rates of alcohol, marijuana, tobacco, and cocaine dependence in 2,755 siblings of 1,212 subjects who met *DSM-III-R* (1987) criteria for alcohol dependence and the Feighner criteria for definite alcoholism. The comparison sample consisted of 217 normal subjects and 254 siblings. For siblings of alcohol-dependent probands, the rates of alcohol, marijuana, cocaine, and tobacco dependence were significantly elevated compared to siblings of nonalcohol-dependent probands. For example, 56.7%, 43.3%, and 61% of the male siblings of alcohol-dependent probands were also marijuana, cocaine, or tobacco dependent, compared to 15.2%, 13.7%, and 35.7% of the siblings of nonalcohol dependents, respectively. The family and twin study results clearly show that there is a common genetic and shared environmental liability underlying all forms of substance use, and use of one substance does indeed increase the risk for using others.

THE ADDICTIVE PERSONALITY?

Clinical research repeatedly identifies antisocial personality disorder as a major risk factor for alcohol dependence (e.g., Lewis & Bucholz, 1991; Sher & Trull, 1994; Strain, 1995). Indeed, scores on personality trait scales such as psychoticism from the Eysenck Personality Questionnaire (EPQ-R: Eysenck & Eysenck, 1992) accounted for more of the variance in drinking behavior than a positive family history for drinking (e.g., Conrod, Peterson, & Pihl, 1997). Similarly, McGue, Slutske, Taylor, and Iacono (1997) reported that the higher order dimensions of negative emotionality, lack of constraint, and behavioral disinhibition from the Multidimensional Personality Questionnaire were able to differentiate between nonalcoholic control and alcoholic samples.

Heath et al. (1997) examined the association of personality (EPQ-R and TPQ), psychopathology (lifetime Axis I disorders), and *DSM-III-R* (1987) alcohol-dependence risk in females and males. In women, the strongest associations with alcohol dependence were found for history of childhood conduct disorder (odds ratio: OR = 4.6), lifetime history of major depression (OR = 2.1), EPQ extraversion (OR = 1.6), and neuroticism (OR = 1.6) scores in the highest quartiles, as well as scores on social nonconformity (OR > 1.9). On the TPQ, only scores above the 75% percentile on novelty seeking (OR = 1.6) were associated with alcohol dependence. Predictors of alcohol dependence in men were very similar to those found in women, with the genders differing only in terms of magnitude. The association with history of childhood conduct disorder is somewhat lower in males (OR = 1.9), but greater on EPQ neuroticism (OR = 1.9).

Phenotypic research has generally shown that personality variables unrelated to antisocial personality appear to have little relationship to alcoholism. For example, Schuckit (1983) showed that EPQ-R extraversion and neuroticism scores for nonalcoholic men with a close alcoholic relative did not differ from those of control subjects. Subsequently, Schuckit, Klein, Twitchell, and Smith (1994) showed that EPQ-R neuroticism and extraversion scores assessed nearly a decade later did not differ in a group of men who developed alcoholic dependence after initial testing.

The Genetic Basis of Antisocial Personality and Alcohol Problems

Behavioral genetic research has shown that the relationship between substance use and antisocial personality has a genetic basis. A small early study of general population twins reported the genetic correlation (r_G) between measures of alcohol problems and measures of childhood antisocial behavior at .54, with adult antisocial behavior estimated at .75 (Grove et al., 1990). Recently, Slutske et al. (2002) estimated the genetic correlations between alcohol and personality traits using a large sample of twins from Australia. They measured alcohol dependence, positive emotionality (derived from the TPQ reward dependence and EPQ-R Extraversion scales), negative emotionality (TPQ harm avoidance and EPQ-R neuroticism), and behavioral undercontrol (TPQ novelty seeking, EPQ-R psychoticism, and reverse coded EPQ-R lie scales), a dimension representing antisocial behavior.

They reported that behavioral undercontrol shared a significant proportion of its genetic liability with alcohol dependence (male r_G = .53; 95% CI: .38–.67; female r_G = .71; 95% CI: .56–.86) and childhood conduct disorder (male r_G = .59; 95% CI: .45–.72; female r_G = .59; 95% CI: .50–.85). Because of the strong relationship between behavioral undercontrol and childhood conduct disorder, these two variables were combined and the proportion of genetic covariation in common alcohol dependence was estimated. The results were striking. This composite variable accounted for 85% (95% CI: 54%–100%) in males and 93% (95% CI: 59%–100%) in females!

Jang et al. (2000) found that specific antisocial personality traits were related to alcohol misuse. Antisocial personality has been defined by several subtraits: sensation seeking, recklessness, callousness, impulsivity, remorselessness, sadism, interpersonal hostility, interpersonal violence, juvenile antisocial behavior, and failure to adopt social norms in the DAPP measure. The genetic and environmental correlations revealed that specific antisocial features had more salience in alcohol misuse (see Fig. 7.1). The highest genetic correlations were found with conduct problems, grandiosity, attention seeking, and narcissistic behavior. In contrast, stimulus seeking, callousness, and rejection sensitivity had only a modest genetic relationship with alcohol misuse.

Substance Use and Psychopathology

Alcohol abuse and dependence (indeed, virtually any kind of substance abuse) is observed in a large proportion of psychiatric patients. This raises the question of

Scales	r_P	r_G	r_E
Stimulus Seeking			
Sensation Seeking	**0.25**	**0.33**	**0.19**
Recklessness	**0.31**	**0.45**	**0.20**
Impulsivity	**0.36**	**0.45**	**0.31**
Callousness			
Contemptuousness	**0.15**	**0.19**	**0.12**
Egocentrism	**0.21**	**0.19**	**0.23**
Exploitation	**0.18**	**0.19**	**0.16**
Interpersonal irresponsibility	**0.19**	**0.24**	**0.15**
Lack of empathy	**0.10**	0.10	**0.11**
Remorselessness	**0.15**	**0.31**	0.01
Sadism	**0.29**	**0.36**	**0.22**
Rejection			
Rigid cognitive style	**0.16**	**0.27**	0.09
Judgmental	**0.11**	**0.20**	0.05
Interpersonal hostility	**0.25**	**0.41**	**0.12**
Dominance	0.04	0.03	0.04
Conduct problems			
Interpersonal violence	**0.32**	**0.78**	**0.33**
Juvenile antisocial behavior	**0.38**	**0.67**	**0.40**
Failure to adopt social norms	**0.40**	**0.85**	0.03
Suspiciousness			
Hypervigilance	**0.13**	**0.37**	**0.14**
Suspiciousness	**0.13**	**0.60**	0.08
Narcissism			
Need for adulation	**0.15**	**0.55**	-0.07
Attention seeking	**0.21**	**0.87**	-0.02
Grandiosity	**0.18**	**0.88**	-0.08

FIG. 7.1. Phenotypic (r_p), genetic (r_G), and nonshared environmental (r_E) correlations, 95% confidence intervals between alcohol misuse and DAPP-DQ dissocial and facet scales. N_{MZ} = 324 pairs; N_{DZ} = 335 pairs; boldface = significant at $p < 0.05$; r_p is based on 659 subjects in which one member of each pair was randomly selected. Adapted from "Personality Disorder Traits, Family Environment, and Alcohol Misuse: A Multivariate Behavioral Genetic Analysis," by K. L. Jang, P. A. Vernon, and W. J. Livesley, 2000, *Addiction, 95*, p. 881. Copyright 2000 by Elsevier Science. Adapted with permission.

whether specific forms of substance abuse are more prevalent with particular psychopathologies. For example, is nicotine dependence more prevalent among schizophrenics? Is alcohol dependence more prevalent among patients diagnosed with major depressive disorder? Broadening the issue a little, the literature has shown that initiation and dependence are influenced by different genetic factors, raising the question of whether different psychopathologies differentially influence risk for initiation, persistence, abuse, and dependence.

Kendler, Neale, et al. (1999) examined this question by estimating the predictive validity of a wide range of risk factors for smoking initiation and nicotine dependence. The risk factor variables included religiosity, neuroticism and extraversion, altruism, dependency, mastery, powerlessness, locus of control, *DSM-III-R* (1987) lifetime history of major depression, GAD, panic disorder, phobias, bulimia nervosa, and alcohol dependence. Among the demographic variables, a regression analysis selected years of education (fewer), low levels of personal religious devotion (all OR < 1.0), and divorce (OR = 2.51) as the best predictors of smoking initiation. The best predictors of nicotine dependence were years of education and individual income (all OR < 1.0). Most of the personality variables were also associated with increased risk for initiation and dependence (OR range 0.84–1.31). Like the demographic and personality factors, psychopathology was also found to be associated with a statistically significant but modest increase in risk. For smoking initiation, major depression (OR = 1.89), GAD (OR = 1.97), panic disorder (OR = 3.51), phobias (OR = 1.54), problem drinking (OR = 4.11), and alcohol dependence (OR = 5.63) emerged as significant risks. For nicotine dependence, major depression (OR = 2.11), GAD (OR = 2.28), problem drinking (OR = 1.86), and alcohol dependence (OR = 2.47) emerged as significant. Merikangas and Avenevoli (2000), in their family study of substance use, also found increased rates of lifetime substance use with premorbid psychopathology among children of probands. The odds ratios are presented in Fig. 7.2. They write that the clinical significance of the comorbidity between certain forms of psychopathology and substance use disorders provides new opportunities to identify targets of prevention. Because effective treatments do exist for many of the primary psychiatric disorders, treatment of the underlying disorder may serve to prevent the development of substance abuse.

ENVIRONMENTAL EFFECTS

The previous section concentrated on the role of genetic effects. The remainder of this chapter examines research that has identified the environmental effects important in substance use. One variable that continually appears in the literature is family environment.

In the substance abuse literature, the Family Environment scale (FES: Moos & Moos, 1994) is frequently used to measure specific aspects of the family environment. This retrospective scale measures a person's perceptions of the family environment. Research with the FES and alcoholism has yielded consistent phenotypic relationships. Barry and Fleming (1990) found that subjects with a family history of

Premorbid Psychiatric Disorder	Substance Use Adjusted Odds Ratios (95% CIs)		
	Use	Abuse	Dependence
Affective	0.6 (0.2-2.1)	1.7(0.6-4.8)	3.2 (1.1-9.3)
Conduct	4.2 (0.5-38.4)	6.0(1.7-21.4)	6.0 (1.7-20.9)
Oppositional	4.2 (1.0-17.8)	3.3 (0.8-12.7)	4.1 (1.1-14.7)
ADHD	0.9 (0.3-2.7)	2.0 (0.5-7.8)	3.6 (1.0-13.5)
Anxiety	0.9 (0.3-2.2)	1.9 (0.7-5.0)	5.5 (1.80-16.3)
Any disorder	1.3 (0.6-3.0)	3.0 (1.0-9.1)	5.7 (1.4-22.7)

FIG. 7.2.   Yale Family Study: Comorbidity of lifetime substance use and premorbid psychopathology among offspring (N = 203). Adapted from "Implications of Genetic Epidemiology for the Prevention of Substance Use Disorders," by K. R. Merikangas and S. Avenevoli, 2000, *Addictive Behaviors, 25*, p. 814. Copyright 2000 by Elsevier Science. Adapted with permission.

alcohol abuse reported their families of origin to be lower in cohesion (the degree of commitment, help, and support family members provide to each other), but higher in conflict (amount of openly expressed anger) than subjects who do not have a family history of alcohol abuse.

Wilson, Bell, and Arredondo (1995) reported the same results in a later study, but also found that scores on intellectual-cultural orientation (levels of interest in political, intellectual, and cultural activities), activity (amount of participation in social and recreational activities), and organization (degree of importance of clear structure in planning family activities and responsibilities) were significantly lower in subjects who had a family history of alcohol abuse. When the samples were divided by gender, females reported their families as lower in achievement orientation (how much school or work are cast into a competitive or achievement framework) and intellectual-cultural orientation, and higher in expressiveness (the extent to which family members are encouraged to directly express feelings). Harvey and Dodd (1995) used the FES to compare the family environments of a sample of sixth-grade children of alcoholics and children of nonalcoholics. They found that the best predictors of early experimentation with alcohol, drugs, and tobacco were again conflict and cohesion.

Religiosity

A recent study of alcohol use initiation by Koopman, Slutske, Van Baal, and Boomsma (1999) suggests that religion moderates the genetic variability in alcohol use. They measured participants' initiation of alcohol use and whether they were currently active in church, or reported they were religious but were not active in church in a sample of Dutch adolescent twin pairs (MZ males = 327, MZ females = 457, DZ males = 284, DZ females = 356, DZ opposite-sex = 543). They found that the magnitude of the genetic influences on risk of alcohol use initiation was higher in families without a religious upbringing than in families with it. They also reported that, among religious males, the heritability of alcohol use was lower than in nonreligious males: $h^2_A = 25\%$ (95% CI: 7%–48%), $c^2 = 67\%$ (46%–82%), and $e^2 = 7\%$ (3%–16%) versus $h^2_A = 40\%$ (95% CI: 5%–69%), $c^2 = 47\%$ (20%–76%), and $e^2 = 13\%$ (6%–26%). It should be noted that the difference in h^2_A was not statistically significant, but was consistent with a trend that supports the idea that religiosity moderates genetic effects. However, among religious females, the heritability was not significant: $h^2_A = 0\%$ (95% CI: 0%–17%), $c^2 = 88\%$ (72%–92%), and $e^2 = 12\%$ (7%–19%), versus nonreligious: $h^2_A = 39\%$ (95% CI: 14%–66%), $c^2 = 56\%$ (29%–78%), and $e^2 = 5\%$ (2%–11%).

This study also found that an important aspect of antisocial personality, behavioral disinhibition, was significantly correlated with alcohol use ($r = .46$ in males and $r = .41$ in females) and that the heritability of behavioral disinhibition was significantly greater among those who reported less religious involvement. Koopman et al. (1999) concluded that genetic influences on disinhibited behavior (which includes heavier and problematic alcohol use) among more religious individuals are attenuated because their decision on how to behave is based less on personal choice and more on family circumstances or religious proscriptions (p. 446). Thus, religious upbringing reduces the impact of genotype on disinhibited behavior as well as on initiation.

It is important to remember that variables such as religiosity may be acting as a proxy for other variables. For example, a study by Heath et al. (1997) found that religious practices acted as a protective factor against alcohol dependence. Specifically, women reporting a religious affiliation of "other Protestant" or "at least weekly church attendance" were associated with decreased risk for alcoholism (OR = 0.64 and 0.44, respectively). In contrast, reporting no religious affiliation was associated with an increased risk (OR = 1.98). No associations were found with educational level, twin zygosity, or marital status. In males, alcoholism rates were significantly elevated in those reporting a Catholic religious affiliation (OR = 1.69), but the risk was significantly reduced in those with a university education (OR = 0.59), in those born prior to 1930 (OR = 0.32), and in those reporting "at least weekly church attendance" (OR = 0.49).

Is there something about being Catholic that influences alcoholism? The answer is likely "no." Heath et al. (1997) suggested that Catholicism is probably best considered a proxy variable for ethnicity, specifically Australians of Irish ancestry, which may in part reflect underlying genetic differences and may explain why it is associated with increased alcoholism risk in the males of this sample. They also reported that c^2 effects accounted for 1% to 3% of the total variance in male and female alcoholism, and concluded that, within this sample, shared experiences including parental drinking and alcoholism, growing up in the same family and in the same neighborhood, and attending the same school are not important determinants of sibling resemblance for alcoholism.

Marriage

Heath, Eaves, and Martin (1989) tested whether being married or being in a marriage-like relationship moderates the genetic basis to drinking habits. The study sample was 1,233 MZ and 751 DZ female adult same-sex twin pairs from Australia who were interviewed on the details of total weekly alcohol consumption. This consisted of reports measured in standard drink sizes (7 oz [207 ml] of beer, 4 oz [118 ml] of wine, 1 oz [30 ml] of spirits) for each day of the preceding 7-day week. Current marital status information was obtained: unmarried (single, separated, divorced, or widowed) or married (married or living together). The twins were further subdivided into two age cohorts: younger adults (30 years and younger) and older adults (31 years and older).

To test for gene-environment interaction effects, they estimated the magnitude of h^2_A, c^2, and e^2 conditional on environmental exposure: married versus unmarried status. In a model where there are no gene-environment interaction effects, estimates of h^2_A, c^2, and e^2 should not significantly differ between married and unmarried twins. If gene-environment interaction effects are present, it is expected that estimates of h^2_A, c^2, and e^2 should vary significantly between married and unmarried twins. Their results were clear: Marital status does moderate (decreases) genetic influences on alcohol consumption. In the younger adult cohort, h^2_A for unmarried twins was 60% compared to married twins, where $h^2_A = 31\%$. In the older adult cohort, h^2_A for unmarried twins was estimated at 76%, whereas in married twins h^2_A was 59%. When the older and younger cohorts were combined, h^2_A was 77% for unmarried twins and 59% for married twins.[1]

Urban and Rural Settings

Like religious upbringing or marital status, another variable that consistently emerges as important is where one lives. The most recent studies of the effects of socioregional variation (e.g., urban vs. rural living) in the context of gene-environ-

---

[1] Heath et al. (1989) were quick to caution that even if significant differences were seen in estimates of h^2_A, c^2, or e^2 between married and unmarried twins, this does not automatically imply that gene-environment interaction effects are present. Differences in heritability estimates could be attributable to differences in the average levels of alcohol consumption between married and unmarried groups. Average differences are usually accompanied by greater variances and this could translate into differences in h^2_A, c^2, or e^2. A second possibility is that there are group differences in the amount of random error between married and unmarried groups. The third alternative explanation for the results is the degree of social interaction between spouses. For example, heavy drinking by one spouse encourages heavy drinking in the other. Heath et al. noted that it is presently unclear if heavy drinkers prefer to marry other heavy drinkers (e.g., assortative mating) or if this effect is due to reciprocal environmental influences between spouses. The presence of either effect would increase the variation in consumption for the married group relative to the unmarried group, leading to differences in estimates of h^2_A, c^2, or e^2 that have nothing to do with the effect of the environment on the genotype. They tested for these potential biases and concluded with some confidence that the differences in heritability are due to gene-environment interaction effects.

ment interaction were conducted in Finland. The "FinnTwin" projects are population-based studies of several consecutive birth cohorts of Finnish twins and their drinking habits (cf. Rose, Kaprio, Winter, Koskenvuo, & Viken, 1999).

One of the earliest studies examined whether urban versus rural living influenced abstinence. Rose et al. (1999) analyzed data from 2,711 pairs of known zygosity identified from five consecutive birth-cohorts. The age of the twins at the time of this study was 16 and they completed a general questionnaire on health habits and lifestyle. Twins from greater Helsinki (urban) and northern Finland (rural) were first examined for overall resemblance on alcohol use; abstinence from alcohol to age 16 was found to be largely due to shared family (c^2) influences. Twin resemblance for abstinence over the entire sample was very high, with $r_{MZF} = .97$ and $r_{DZF} = .87$; similarly, $r_{MZM} = .90$ and $r_{DZM} = .82$. However, the twin concordances changed significantly when the twins were separated by where they lived. For example, MZM and DZM concordance for abstinence in greater Helsinki was estimated at .87 and .50 (Falconer's $h^2_B = .73$), respectively, whereas in northern Finland, the MZM and DZM concordances were .77 and .77 (Falconer's $h^2_B = 0.0$). Similar results were reported for females: MZF and DZF concordances in Helsinki were .82 and .44 (Falconer's $h^2_B = 75\%$), whereas in northern Finland, the concordances were .83 and .78 respectively, yielding a Falconer's estimate of h^2_B at about 10%.

Rose et al. (1999) concluded that their results were consistent with the idea that environmental effects modulate the influences of siblings and parents on adolescent abstinence. They noted that the effects may be developmentally transient and disappear as the subjects age. The exact nature of the environmental effects needs closer examination. Area of residence is likely a proxy variable for other effects. They suggested that the Finnish urban-rural divide represents several environmental variables, such as ease of access to liquor stores, regional variation in levels of community and familial control of adolescent drinking, and availability of extended networks of peers. Urban and rural adolescents in Finland experience different exposure to public drinking and intoxication and there are well-documented historical and regional differences in religious values and religious behavior.

In another study, the effect of residency on alcohol use over 2 years was studied (Rose, Dick, Viken, Pulkkinen, & Kaprio, 2001). In this study, data on drinking frequency were obtained from adolescents at ages 16, 17, and 18.5. Unlike the previous study, which focused on abstinence, this report analyzed all levels of alcohol use (e.g., daily, twice a week, once a week, twice a month, about once a month, about once every 2 months, three to four times a year, once a year or less, never). Heritability analyses over the three ages showed that genetic factors influencing drinking patterns increased over the 30-month period. At ages 16, 17, and 18.5, the h^2_A for drinking frequency was reported to account for 33% (95% CI: 26%–43%), 49% (95% CI: 39%–61%), and 50% (95% CI: 39%–63%) of the total variance; c^2 influences accounted for 37% (95% CI: 28%–45%), 20% (95% CI: 10%–29%), 14% (95% CI: 3%–22%), respectively, with e^2 accounting for 29% (95% CI: 21%–37%), 30% (95% CI: 22%–38%), and 36% (95% CI: 28%–45%).

When the estimates were crossed with area of residency, a clear genotype-by-environment interaction was detected. Genetic factors assumed a larger role among adolescents residing in urban areas, whereas shared environmental influences were more important in rural settings. Another surprising finding is that urban and rural settings appear to moderate genetic and environmental influences on adolescent drinking without altering abstinence rates among nondrinkers or drinking frequency among nonabstinent adolescents. This suggests that the environmental factors on average levels of drinking are different from the moderating effect of the environment. For example, urban areas may not necessarily encourage adolescents to initiate drinking earlier, to drink more frequently, or to drink greater quantities, but rather provide the opportunities for those who are genetically predisposed to engage in drinking to do so. At the same time, the diversity of the urban environment enables adolescents who abstain from drinking (or drink rarely) to find like-minded and supportive peers. In rural areas, environmental influences tend to cluster between communities, and thus between families, which are then detected as c^2 effects.

SUMMARY

The research reviewed in this chapter shows that alcohol, nicotine, and illicit drug use are substantially heritable. Generally, across general population and clinical samples, heritability estimates range from 45% to 55%. The majority of environmental influence is nonshared in nature. Shared environmental effects appear to account for a significant proportion of the variance (around 15%) only in studies that have ascertained twins in treatment programs. Regarding gender, there is some evidence to suggest that different genetic factors influence male and female substance use problems, and that some of those gender differences are tied to age.

Multivariate genetic analyses have shown that alcohol, nicotine, and several classes of illicit drug use share to some extent a common genetic basis, suggesting that use of one substance will increase the risk for the use of others. However, the use of other substances is not inevitable. Research on gene-environment interaction has consistently identified a number of environmental factors that moderate these genetically-based risks, including family environment (e.g, perceptions of family cohesion), marriage, availability of substances, and religiosity.

Personality factors, particularly those associated with antisocial personality, are associated with increased risk for substance use and abuse. Multivariate genetic analyses suggest that a component of the genetic liability to substance use is shared with these traits. Studies of gene-environment interplay suggest that personality factors appear to increase the risk for substance use by influencing the individual to favor and seek high-risk environments. Another growing body of research is showing that environmental factors moderate genetic propensities to alcoholism. High-risk environments, as shown by the FinnTwin studies, such as urban settings that provide the opportunities (e.g., greater accessibility to liquor) for those with the propensities to engage in drinking or other substance use.

Chapter 8

Schizophrenia and the Psychotic Disorders

The psychotic disorders are probably the most dramatic of the psychiatric conditions, with their prominent delusions, hallucinations, and disorganized speech and behavior. The clarity of the psychotic phenotype makes it an ideal disorder to study from a genetic perspective. Interest in these disorders, especially schizophrenia, has led to some of the most comprehensive theories explaining their development. This chapter examines the behavioral genetic support for the most commonly accepted theory: that schizophrenia is a neurodevelopmental disorder in which a fixed brain lesion in early life interacts with maturational events that occur much later (Weinberger, 1987). This hypothesis is based on the idea that a brain lesion can remain clinically silent until normal developmental processes bring the structures affected by the lesion "on line" (Marenco & Weinberger, 2000).

Support for this model would consist of evidence for: (a) a genetic predisposition for the disorder, (b) influence of environmental phenomena on gene expression at critical times during development, (c) the impact of altered patterns of gene expression on other developmental processes and subsequent behavior, and (d) the largely permanent nature of any alterations in gene expression (Lewis & Levitt, 2002). In this chapter, I review some of the recent behavioral genetic research in each of these four areas. Most of the published research is relevant to the first three issues, particularly the first. There is a large amount of molecular genetic literature, a cursory review of which would fill a book, and several excellent reviews of this literature have already been published.

To provide a sample of what has been found, there have been several reports that possible susceptibility genes have been located on chromosomes 6p and 8p (e.g., Moises, Yang, Kristbjarnarson, et al., 1995; Pulver et al., 1995; Schwab et al., 1995; Wang et al., 1994). Replications on chromosome 10p have also been reported

(Faraone et al, 1999; Straub et al., 1998), as well as on 13q (Blouin et al., 1998), 15q (Kaufman et al., 1998), and 22q (Moises, Yang, Li, et al., 1995). Other possible hot spots include the gene encoding for chromogranin B (a protein found in the secretory granules of a wide variety of endocrine and neuroendocrine cells), specifically, marker D20S95 (Kitao et al., 2000), and chromosome 6p24 in the region of D6S309, which neared significance (Bailer et al., 2000). It is interesting to note that results nearing statistical significance are as important as those that actually reach it! The notion of disturbances in glutamate function controlled by the gene GRM4 has received some support (e.g., Ohtsuki, Toru, & Arinami, 2001) as has enzyme function, specifically catechol-o-methyltransferase function and its genes (Chaldee et al., 2001) and human leukocyte antigens (HLA) on chromosome 6p (see Wright, Nimgaonkar, Donaldson, & Murray, 2001, for a review).

For the present, the most important finding to be gleaned from this literature has not been that possible susceptibility genes have been identified, but rather that most cases of schizophrenia are not caused by a single gene of major effect (see also Gottesman, 1991; Tsuang, Stone, & Faraone, 1999, 2001). Single-gene models do not explain the pattern of illness in either families or twins (e.g., MZ concordance rates are less than 100% as would be predicted by this model). Accordingly, this chapter focuses mainly on the twin and family study research to determine what causes this less-than-perfect concordance in the context of the neurodevelopmental model of schizophrenia.

BEHAVIORAL GENETIC EVIDENCE
FOR THE NEURODEVELOPMENTAL MODEL

The Heritable Basis of Schizophrenia

Twin studies have provided ample evidence that there is a genetic basis for schizophrenia. Across studies, this disorder is consistently shown to have the highest heritability, with estimates from 80% or more (see Sullivan, Kendler, & Neale, 2003). These results are consistent not only across different studies, but also across different definitions of schizophrenia. For example, Cardno et al. (1999) estimated the heritability of Research Diagnostic Criteria (RDC), *DSM-III-R* (1987) and ICD-10 (1992) schizophrenia diagnoses and other functional psychoses on a sample of 106 MZ and 118 DZ same-sex twin pairs in which at least one member had a lifetime history of psychosis. The genetic contribution (h^2_B) to the major diagnoses was substantial at 82% to 85%, with nonshared environmental effects accounting for the remainder. Moreover, the heritability estimates for other functional psychoses were also high, ranging from 80% to 87%. The specific results are presented in Fig. 8.1.

The substantial heritability associated with the diagnoses has also been found for the symptoms of schizophrenia. Cardno, Sham, Farmer, Murray, and McGuffin (2002) estimated the heritability of the "first-rank symptoms" in a sample of 224 same-sex twin pairs (106 MZ and 118 DZ). First-rank symptoms included audible

Heritability Estimates of Best-Fitting Model (95% CI)

Diagnoses	h^2		h_d^2	c^2	e^2	
Research Diagnostic Criteria						
Lifetime-ever						
Schizophrenia	0.82	(0.71-0.90)	...	...	0.18	(0.10-0.29)
Schizoaffective	0.85	(0.70-0.94)	...	...	0.15	(0.06-0.30)
Disorders, all						
Manic	0.80	(0.57-0.94)	...	...	0.20	(0.06-0.43)
Depressed	0.87	(0.67-0.97)	...	...	0.13	(0.03-0.33)
Affective psychoses	0.83	(0.72-0.91)	...	...	0.17	(0.09-0.28)
All						
Mania	0.84	(0.69-0.93)	...	...	0.16	(0.07-0.31)
Mania/hypomania	0.87	(0.75-0.95)	...	...	0.13	(0.05-0.25)
Depressive psychosis						
Unspecified functional						
Psychosis						
OPCRIT main-lifetime						
DSM-III-R						
Schizophrenia	0.00	(0.00-0.64)	0.84 (0.19-0.92)	...	0.16	(0.08-0.26)
ICD-10 schizophrenia	0.00	(0.00-0.75)	0.83 (0.07-0.91)	...	0.16	(0.09-0.27)

FIG. 8.1.   Heritability of schizophrenia and other functional psychoses. Adapted from "Heritability Estimates for Psychotic Disorders: The Maudsley Twin Psychosis Series," by A. G. Cardno et al., 1999, *Archives of General Psychiatry, 56*, p. 166. Copyright 1999 by American Medical Association. Adapted with permission.

thoughts, running commentary, third-person auditory hallucination, thought withdrawal, insertion and broadcasting, delusional perception, and delusions of control that included made feelings, made drives, and somatic passivity (Schneider, 1959). The twins were rated on these symptoms and the ratings were totaled. Additive genetic effects (h_A^2) were found to account for 71% (95% CI: 57%–82%) of the total variance with nonshared environmental effects accounting for the remainder ($e^2 = 29\%$: 95% CI: 18%–43%).

The heritable basis of schizophrenia has also been demonstrated using endophenotypes such as brain volume. For example, brain volume data from 15 MZ and 14 DZ twin pairs discordant for schizophrenia were recently published Baaré et al. (2001). Their study began by showing that there were significant differences in brain volume between schizophrenics and a sample of normal controls matched for zygosity, sex, and age. Irrespective of zygosity, the whole brain (2%), parahippocampal (9%), and hippocampal (8%) volumes of discordant twin pairs were smaller compared to healthy twin controls.

Among the discordant pairs, the affected members were found to have smaller brains (2.2%) than their healthy cotwins, who in turn had smaller brains (1%) than controls. Differences in ventricular volumes were also observed. Among all of the discordant twin pairs, the affected twin's lateral ventricles were larger (14.4%) compared to their nonschizophrenic twins. However, within the discordant DZ pairs, the lateral and third ventricular volumes were much larger compared to the healthy cotwins (60.6% and 56.6% larger, respectively). Thus, consistent with a genetic hypothesis, the unaffected cotwins occupy an intermediate position between their ill siblings and the healthy controls. Examination of MZ-to-DZ twin correlations for discordant pairs also provides support for the genetic basis of brain volume. The MZ exceeds the DZ correlation for all brain structures except the parahippocampal gyrus, yielding Falconer heritability estimates (h^2_B) that range from a low of 36% (volume of third ventricle) to 100% (hippocampal volume), with a median heritability of 97%.

The similarity of the heritability estimates for the symptoms of schizophrenia, schizophrenia diagnoses, and the other functional psychoses suggests that psychosis exists on a single, genetically based continuum. However, tests of this hypothesis by Cannon, Kaprio, Loennqvist, Huttunen, and Koskenvuo (1998) suggest another scenario. Their sample consisted of 1,180 MZ male, 1,315 MZ female, 2,765 DZ male and 2,613 DZ female, and 163 DZ opposite-sex twin pairs from Finland. All were screened for schizophrenia using ICD-8 (1967) and DSM-III-R (1987) criteria. The twins were assigned to one of three categories (most to least severe): (a) schizophrenia, (b) affective psychosis, or (c) other psychoses (e.g., paranoid psychosis, reactive psychosis, or unspecified psychosis). These diagnostic categories led to four different groupings that reflected a single continuum of illness: (a) schizophrenia only, (b) schizophrenia and affective psychosis, (c) schizophrenia with other psychosis, and (d) schizophrenia, affective, and other psychosis. This ranking along a single continuum of liability would be supported if the twin correlations associated with each group did not differ significantly. Contrary to expectation, they found that the MZ correlation for the schizophrenia-only group was significantly greater than that of other groups, indicating that the genetic composition of the schizophrenia-only group changes when twins with other psychotic disorders are included, thus rejecting the idea that affective and other psychoses fall somewhere between no diagnosis and schizophrenia.

Cannon et al. (1998) also found no evidence of gender-based genetic differences in schizophrenia. They estimated the heritability (h^2_B) of a combined sample of male and female schizophrenics at 83%, with nonshared environmental effects accounting for the remainder of the variance ($e^2 = 17\%$). When the analyses were repeated by gender, for males: $h^2_B = 83\%$ with e^2 accounting for the remainder (17%). Among women the estimates were similar: $h^2_B = 85\%$ and $e^2 = 15\%$. Subsequent sex-limitation analyses detected no gender-specific genetic or environmental effects.

Franzek and Beckmann (1998) reported similar results based on a sample of twins in which at least one member of each pair was diagnosed with schizophrenia spectrum psychoses. This sample consisted of 45 twin pairs (22 MZ and 23 DZ). The MZ and DZ concordance rates for *DSM-III-R* (1987) schizophrenia were 87.5% and 25.0% respectively. For a broader definition including schizophreniform, schizoaffective, and delusional (paranoid) disorder and psychotic disorder not otherwise specified, the MZ concordance dropped to 47.1%, whereas the DZ remained steady at 30.8%. These results suggest that the heritability of schizophrenia remains high, but as the definition is broadened, the aetiological basis changes radically.

Franzek and Beckmann (1998) found the same pattern of results when the definition of schizophrenia was changed to Leonhard's (1979) diagnostic system which differs from the *DSM* in that a diagnosis can only be made if all of the clinical features fit; that is, the diagnosis cannot be made if the characteristic symptoms are absent. The *DSM* system, on the other hand, makes a diagnosis based on the presence of some or all of the specific symptoms of a symptom cluster. Leonhard's system specifies three types of psychoses: unsystematic schizophrenia, systematic schizophrenia, and cycloid psychoses.

Leonhard's (1979) cycloid psychosis runs a phasic and prognostically favorable long-term course that is similar to manic-depressive disease. Complete remission and absence of residual symptoms are characteristic of this disorder. The symptoms defining this diagnosis are found across several *DSM-III-R* (1987) diagnoses, ranging from bipolar mood disorders with psychotic features to strictly defined schizophrenia. Unsystematic schizophrenias are slightly more severe and circumscribed. The diagnostic criteria are similar to those of cycloid psychosis, but are differentiated by residual states of varying severity. Franzek and Beckmann (1998) noted that for the most part they resemble the *DSM-III-R* definition of schizophrenia. Leonhard's systematic schizophrenia is described as beginning insidiously and running a chronic, progressive course without remission. It is considered untreatable. The MZ concordance for cycloid psychoses was estimated at 38.5 and the DZ concordance at 36.4. Using the more severe forms of the disorder, the MZ concordance for unsystematic schizophrenia was 88.9%, compared to the DZ concordance of 25.0%. Unfortunately, none of the MZ twins in the present sample met the diagnosis for systematic schizophrenia, so the concordance rate could not be estimated. These results also suggest that different forms of psychosis are aetiologically distinct. Interestingly, Franzek and Beckmann noted that birth complications were present in 84% of the twins with a cycloid psychosis, a much greater rate than that of twins with other diagnoses.

A study by Beckmann, Franzek, and Stober (1996) also found evidence that the psychoses do not fall along a single continuum of liability. This study recruited a sample of 139 probands who met *DSM-III-R* (1987) criteria for catatonic schizophrenia, and who were reclassified as suffering from either "systematic catatonia" (83 probands) and "periodic catatonia" (56 probands) using Leonhard's (1979) clinical dichotomy. The study also included 543 of their first-degree relatives. Systematic catatonia is described as beginning insidiously and running a chronically progressive course without remission. In contrast, periodic catatonia is described as typically intermittent and bipolar with hyperkinetic and akinetic states. It is characterized by impulsive behavior as well as depression, expansive or irritable mood swings, and delusions and hallucinations that are present, but not prominent. Symptoms usually disappear during remission of the disorder. Beckmann et al. found little evidence of familial aggregation for systematic catatonia, with the morbidity risk among first-degree relatives estimated at a modest 4.6%. In contrast, the risk for periodic catatonia was 26.9%, suggesting that systematic catatonia is a sporadic form of schizophrenia, whereas periodic catatonia aggregates in families in a manner consistent with a major gene effect.

Even the first-rank symptoms of schizophrenia appear to be differentially heritable. Loftus, Delisi, and Crow (2000) recruited 103 sibling pairs in which one member had a primary diagnosis of *DSM-III-R* (1987) schizophrenia or schizoaffective disorder. These siblings were rated on all first-rank symptoms and these ratings were subjected to factor analysis. Two orthogonal dimensions were extracted. The first factor accounted for approximately 50% of the total variance and was marked by thought broadcasting, thought insertion, thought withdrawal, and delusions of control reflecting anomalies in the generation of speech from thought. The second (accounting for approximately 17% of the total variance) was marked by third-person hallucinations, running commentary, and thought echo. Only the sibling correlation on the first factor was significant ($r = .21$); the sibling correlation on the second factor was near zero ($r = .04$), which indicates that the factors are differentially familial. The results also suggest that the symptoms defining the first factor may represent the heritable core of schizophrenia. It is important to note that this study is based on a family study design and cannot distinguish genetic from possibly competing nongenetic sources of variance.

In summary, the twin research has provided substantial evidence that schizophrenia and other functional psychoses have a significant heritable basis. The data also suggest that these predispositions are largely unique to each disorder. They do not support the hypothesis that these disorders are caused by a single gene of large effect; rather, psychotic disorders are polygenic and multifactorial in nature. The multifactorial nature of these disorders brings us to the second part of this chapter, which focuses on the environmental factors important in the development of schizophrenia.

Environmental Influences

According to a neurodevelopmental model of schizophrenia, gene expression may be influenced or triggered by environmental phenomena during a specific period of ontogeny. These phenomena affect the production or function of protein products that in turn play an essential role in brain function, resulting in an altered course of development that drives the system toward a critical threshold for the disorder (Lewis & Levitt, 2002). Tsuang (2001) recently identified from the literature a number of environmental risk factors that have been shown to cause neurodevelopmental errors during gestation: season of birth, urban density (likely a proxy variable for urban environment caused by excessive noise, pollution, crime, and other negative social factors), and viral infections (e.g., influenza and Coxackie B meningitis of the central nervous system during the pre- or perinatal period).

Pregnancy and delivery complications have also been implicated, such as malnutrition during fetal life, extreme prematurity, and hypoxia or ischemia that may affect brain volume (see Dalman, Alleback, Cullberg, Grunewald, & Koster, 1999). For example, McNeil, Cantor-Graae, and Weinberger (2000) measured the brain volumes of 22 MZ twin pairs discordant for schizophrenia. They found that the affected twin consistently had smaller left and right hippocami, larger left lateral ventricles, and larger third ventricles compared to the unaffected twin. They also found that the relatively small left and right hippocampi, larger right lateral ventricle, and larger total ventricle size were significantly related to labor-delivery complications, especially prolonged labor as opposed to pregnancy complications or minor physical abnormalities.

Another important environmental factor is the level of family functioning. Wahlberg et al. (1997) showed that in a sample of 58 adoptees at high genetic risk for schizophrenia (their biological mothers had been hospitalized for schizophrenia at some point in their lives) appear to have been *protected* by healthy rearing-family environment and were more often psychiatrically disturbed when reared in dysfunctional families compared to 96 control adoptees (whose risk for schizophrenia equaled the population risk). These results are interesting because they suggest that schizophrenia can be prevented.

In this study, vulnerability to schizophrenia was assessed using the Index of Primitive Thoughts, based on the Rorschach inkblot test. This test evaluates the adequacy of individual cognitive function based on a person's responses to the inkblots. The categories of thought disorder are "contamination" (when incompatible percepts are fused and attributed in the same blot area), "confabulation" (inappropriate attribution of a small area to a larger area, e.g., when the whole inkblot is seen as a snake because a small portion looks like a snake head), and "fabulized combination" (two precepts are combined because of contiguity, resulting in a precept that does not occur in nature, such as a "rabbit with bat wings"). In short, the scale detects the developmentally lowest levels of cognitive functioning.

The functionality of the adoptive family environment was indexed by level of communication deviance. Communication deviance is conceptualized as the understandability of discourse, specifically, the degree to which language production is ambiguous and hard to follow. This was assessed in the adoptive parents by scoring their responses to Rorschach protocols for: (a) ambiguous and inconsistent references ("That is the same shape as the other one we had a while ago, only it's in color"), (b) responses in a negative form ("It doesn't look like a sheep"), (c) extraneous questions and remarks ("Could a person be affected by vaccination?"), (d) uncorrected remarks ("But I mean—and I'm talking about the past"), and (e) partial disqualification ("Like a couple of characters doing a dance, dressed alike. More like dogs than people. They don't look like any particular kind of dog, and they don't exactly look like monkeys. They're just sort of figures created by this ink" (Wahlberg et al., 1997, p. 357).

When the proportion of thought-disordered responses of the high-risk and control adoptees were crossed with the levels of communication deviance in the adoptive parents, a clear gene-environment interaction was found (see Fig. 8.2). The odds ratio for high scores on thought disorders as a function of the interaction of genetic risk and communication deviance was estimated at 2.00 (95% CI: 1.14–3.50). In more practical terms, Wahlberg et al. (1997) showed that the interaction of genetic risk and communication deviance resulted in a 12.64% (95% CI: 2.22%–23.07%) difference in risk for thought disorders.

An important implication of Wahlberg et al.'s (1997) results is their refutation of the notion of a "schizophrenogenic" family environment, in which a sufficiently dysfunctional rearing family could generate schizophrenia in almost anyone. This is clearly not the case as low-risk adoptees show no increase in

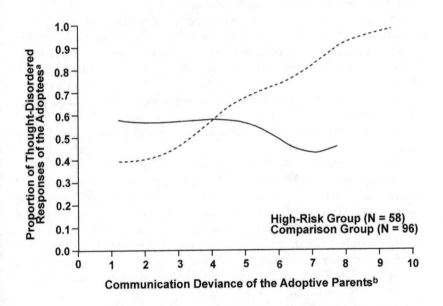

a Proportion of adoptees whose scores on the Index of Primitive Thought were 1 or higher.
b Number of instances of communication deviance (defined in text) per individual Rorschach test.

FIG. 8.2. From "Gene-Environment Interaction in Vulnerability to Schizophrenia: Findings From the Finnish Adoptive Family Study of Schizophrenia," by K. E. Wahlberg et al., 1997, *American Journal of Psychiatry, 154,* p. 358. Copyright 1997 by American Psychiatric Publishing, Inc. Reprinted with permission.

scores of disordered thought with increasing levels of communication deviance in adoptive parents.

Another recent study also dispelled the myth of the schizophrenogenic family, suggesting that family environment can prevent the development of schizophrenia in high-risk individuals. Tienari et al. (2004) demonstrated this using an adoption design to test whether the rate of schizophrenia spectrum disorder differed between high-risk children (whose biological mothers were diagnosed with the disorder) and low-risk children (who had no family history of the disorder) raised in adoptive family environments that differed in levels of functioning. The sample consisted of 303 adopted-away offspring of mother with *DSM-III-R* (1987) schizophrenia spectrum disorders from Finland. The authors developed a scale of family functioning called the Oulun PerheArviontiSkaala (OPAS), or in English, the "Oulu Family Rating scale." The OPAS was developed by drawing items and scales from several existing measures of the family environment as well as by developing new scales that tap major ideas and theories thought to be relevant to the families of schizophrenia. As such, the OPAS assesses generic aspects of family functioning as well as specialized content.

Factor analysis of the scales yielded three domains that described "critical-conflictual relationships," level of "constriction," and "boundary problems." Specifically, the critical-conflictual domain assessed levels of criticism, parent-parent conflict, parent-child conflict, insecurity, lack of empathy, manifest anxiety, inflexibility, and nonacknowledgment. The constriction domain reflected range of affect, rigidity of family structure, passivity, apathy, and lack of humor. Boundary problems assessed the hierarchy versus chaotic structure of the family, levels of individual and generational enmeshment, inadequate daily problem solving, and degree of amorphous communication.

The adoptive families were dichotomized (low vs. high) on these three dimension and the number of the high versus low genetic risk adoptees diagnosed with schizophrenia spectrum disorder were compared. The results clearly showed that adoptees at high genetic risk are more sensitive to problems in the family environment (in all three domains) than low-risk adoptees. The authors also found that high-risk adoptees raised in highly functioning families had significantly fewer schizophrenia spectrum outcomes than high-risk adoptees raised in dysfunctional adoptive families. These results suggest that healthy adoptive families provide a protective influence for high-risk individuals.

There have been other studies suggesting that schizophrenia can be prevented in high-risk individuals. The first requirement for prevention is reliably detecting people who are at high risk. Tsuang, Stone, and Faraone (2002) suggested that the premorbid form of schizophrenia is "schizotaxia" (Meehl, 1962, 1989). Tsuang et al. hypothesized that people with schizotaxia will display moderate deficits on tests such as long-term verbal memory, and attention and executive functions that can be detected by neuropsychological examination scores that are at least two standard deviations below normal in one of these cognitive domains, and at least one standard deviation below normal in a second domain. They also hypothesized that schizotaxic individuals will show moderate levels of negative symptoms for schizophrenia (e.g., by six or more scores of three or higher on Andreasen's [1983] Scale for the Assessment of Negative Symptoms, for example). To put their hypothesis to the test, they identified four individuals with schizotaxia using these diagnostic criteria and treated them with low doses of the antipsychotic medication risperidone which block neurotransmitter receptors, including dopamine and serotonin receptors, in the brain for 6 weeks (Tsuang et al., 1999). All showed marked improvements in attention and mild to moderate reductions in negative symptoms, suggesting that levels of negative symptoms can be treated to prevent possible development of schizophrenia in high-risk families.

Cascade Effects of Altered Development

The third requirement of the neurodevelopmental model is to show that patterns of gene expression affect other developmental processes and subsequent behavior. These effects are also referred to as "cascade effects of altered development" (Lewis & Levitt, 2002). The example given by Lewis and Levitt of this phenomenon is gradual changes in human growth factor expression that lead to subtle changes in glial cell numbers, ultimately affecting synaptic and vascular maturation during adolescence. The behavioral analogue of these molecular events is to show that the genetic and environmental effects underlying one disorder increase the risk for the development of schizophrenia, and vice versa. The presence of such behavioral cascades has been suggested by the long-standing diagnostic categories of schizoaffective and schizotypal personality disorders (i.e., schizotypy) to describe the respective presence of mood and personality in schizophrenia. The significance of the role of personality or mood is readily established by determining if either shares a common aetiology with psychotic symptomology.

Mood and Schizophrenia.   Kendler, Karkowski, and Walsh (1998) showed that affective disorder, and psychotic behavior to some extent, share a common genetic basis, using data from a sample of 343 probands diagnosed with schizophrenia, schizophrenic spectrum disorders, and affective illness, along with 942 of their first-degree relatives from Roscommon County, Ireland. Psychiatric status was determined on the probands and relatives using the SCID for *DSM-III-R* (1987) Axis I disorders and the Structured Interview for Schizotypy for schizophrenia-related personality disorders.

Their first step was to subject all of the ratings to a latent class analysis to sort the symptoms into homogeneous classes of behavior. This analysis yielded six classes of symptoms that were subjected to genetic analysis. The first two classes were "classic schizophrenia," resembling the descriptions of Kraepelin (1919) and Bleuler (1950), and "major depression," with prominent depressive symptoms, nearly absent manic symptoms, and rare psychotic symptoms. The third and fourth classes were "schizophreniform disorder," characterized by levels of hallucinations and delusions similar to those seen in classic schizophrenia, but less severe and with a better outcome; and "bipolar schizomania," characterized by prominent psychotic, manic, and depressive symptoms, with a generally benign course and a favorable outcome. The fifth class was "schizodepression," with symptoms similar to and as prominent as those in classic schizophrenia, but also depressive symptoms as prominent as those seen in major depression. These symptoms were described as having an intermediate course and outcome. The class appears to resemble schizophrenia "a good deal more than typical major depression" (Kendler et al., 1998, p. 494). The final and smallest class described classic features of hebephrenia and was named accordingly. According to the authors, these probands had more pronounced positive thought disorder, inappropriate affect, euphoria, bizarre behavior, distractibility, and recklessness compared to the individuals falling into the classic schizophrenia class.

The genetic analysis estimated the risk for affective and psychotic illness for first-degree relatives of the probands who fell into each of the six classes. Kendler et al. (1998) found significantly increased risk for $DSM-III-R$ (1987) unipolar major depression (morbid risk: 33.7 ± 6.9) in relatives of depressed (Class 2) and schizodrepressed (Class 5) probands (morbid risk for unipolar depression = 25.9 ± 5.2). The risk for $DSM-III-R$ schizophrenia (morbid risk range: 3.8–6.1) and schizophrenia spectrum disorders (morbid risk range: 13.0–19.0) was also increased for the relatives of all classes except major depression (Class 2). Moreover, they found that the risk for $DSM-III-R$ bipolar illness (morbid risk: 4.4 ± 2.3) was increased only in relatives of bipolar-schizomanic probands (Class 4). They concluded that familial vulnerability to psychosis extends across several syndromes and is most pronounced in those with schizophrenia-like symptoms. However, the familial vulnerability to depressive and manic affective illness appears to be somewhat more specific.

These results are mirrored by some typical findings in molecular genetics, in which genes localized for schizophrenia have also been implicated in bipolar disorder. For example, on chromosome 18p, Schwab et al. (1998) reported evidence for linkage to the same markers reportedly linked to bipolar illness (Berrettini et al., 1994). On chromosome 13q32, Detera-Waldleigh et al. (1999) found evidence for linkage of bipolar illness to the same markers for which others (e.g., Blouin et al., 1998) had previously reported evidence for schizophrenia. Despite this genetic overlap, family studies of bipolar probands have in general not found significantly increased rates of schizophrenia in first-degree relatives and vice versa. This literature is neatly summarized by three excellent reviews: Gershon (2000), Berrettini (2000), and Gershon et al. (1998). The idea that there are genes common to ostensibly quite different psychopathologies is a recurrent theme throughout psychiatric genetics. The identification of common genetic liability to affective disorder and schizophrenia, perhaps represented by one of these genes, suggests that what is inherited is a general liability to severe mental illness. An equally important task is to find the genes and possibly the critical environmental influences that distinguish between disorders. The presence or absence of these factors will be key to making an accurate diagnosis and guiding intervention.

Schizotypy. *Schizotypy* is a concept that simultaneously reflects personality aberrations and psychotic symptomology. As a result, the term has come to represent two different disorders in common psychiatric practice. On the one hand, it is commonly considered a variant of schizophrenia linked to the genetic vulnerability of that disorder. This conceptualization focuses on the clinical features shared with schizophrenia, in particular, disordered thinking and lack of deep interpersonal relations identified in the relatives of schizophrenics who exhibited subtle schizophrenia-like psychopathology (Kendler, 1985). This relationship to schizophrenia is recognized in the ICD-10, where schizotypy is classified among the schizophrenias. The other conceptualization emphasizes abnormal personality function, and was developed from clinical observations of relatives of schizophrenics who were consistently described as eccentric or odd, superstitious, and hypersensitive (Kendler, 1985). This conceptualization is codified in the *DSM-IV* (1994) as schizotypal personality disorder (Spitzer, Endicott, & Gibbon, 1979).

So, is schizotypy a form of schizophrenia or a personality disorder? This question has been investigated by estimating the degree to which the symptoms of schizotypy share a common genetic basis with personality or schizophrenia. Recently, work by Linney et al. (2003) suggested that schizotypy is best understood as a form of schizophrenia because the symptoms of schizotypy share a substantial common genetic basis with psychosis-proneness. For this study, a large healthy general population sample of 733 twin pairs from the United Kingdom completed a measure of schizotypy (the Oxford-Liverpool Inventory of Feelings and Experiences or OLIFE: Mason, Claridge, & Jackson, 1995) and a measure of schizophrenic symptomology (the Psychotic Delusions Inventory or PDI: Peters et al., 1999). They found that 42%, 28%, and 49% of the variability in the psychotic features assessed by the PDI were directly attributable to genetic factors common to the OLIFE unusual experiences, cognitive disorganization, and introvertive anhedonia scales.

A study by Berman, Harvey, Smith, and Siever (2000) came to the opposite conclusion by testing whether the structure of schizotypal symptoms derived from the first-degree relatives of schizophrenic patients could be applied to personality-disordered patients. Support for the hypothesis that schizotypy and personality disorder are related would be obtained if the pattern of schizotypal symptoms could explain the symptom patterns present in personality-disordered patients. Schizotypy was assessed in a sample of 172 (67 male and 105 female) nonpsychotic first-degree relatives of schizophrenia patients. They were assessed via first-degree interviews for Axis I disorders, using the Comprehensive Assessment of Symptoms and History (SADS), and for Axis II disorders using the Structured Interview for Diagnosing *DSM-III-R* (1987) Personality Disorders (SIDP). Integrated into the SIDP were several additional questions assessing schizotypy (Kendler, Lieberman, & Walsh, 1989; Silverman et al., 1998).

Confirmatory factor analysis found that the symptoms of schizotypy were organized into three factors. Berman et al. (2000) called these factors the "Disorganization Three Factor Model." The first factor described cognitive-perceptual difficulties, including (factor loadings in parentheses): ideas of reference (.72), magical thinking (.62), unusual perceptual experiences (.52), and suspiciousness (.52). The second factor described interpersonal problems with the symptoms of constricted affect (.76), no close friends (.74), social anxiety (.48), and suspiciousness (.27). The third factor described behavioral disorganization such as odd behavior (.52) and odd speech (.55). The three factors showed a fair degree of overlap, with factor intercorrelations ranging from .52 to .77. This model was then applied to a sample of 143 patients diagnosed with at least one personality disorder. The results showed that these three factors could not be fitted to the personality disorder sample, suggesting that the structure of schizotypal traits in relatives of schizophrenics is not identical to that of personality disorder patients.

Battaglia et al. (1999) obtained similar results, but also showed that schizotypy could be broken down into three aetiologically distinct disorders. Symptoms of schizotypy were assessed using the Structured Clinical Interview for Diagnosing DSM-III-R (1987) Personality Disorders (SCID-PD) in a small sample of 59 twin pairs (23 MZ and 36 DZ same-sex pairs) recruited from the general population of Milan, Italy. Using latent class analysis, they extracted three classes of schizotypal symptomology and estimated the heritability of each. The first latent class was characterized by constricted affect-aloofness and off appearance or odd behavior, with $h^2_A = 49\%$ and $e^2 = 51\%$. The second class was characterized by a degree of interpersonal sensitivity, expressed in the form of social anxiety and ideas of reference, and to a lesser extent suspiciousness. This class was found to be wholly environmental, with $h^2_A = 0.00\%$, $c^2 = 0.00\%$, and $e^2 = 100\%$. Magical thinking, unusual perceptual experiences, and suspiciousness characterized the third latent class. Biometric twin analyses estimated h^2_A at 42% and e^2 at 58%. The authors wrote that the presence of suspiciousness appears to be exclusive to the classes that best describe schizotypal personality disorder, as opposed to schizotypal schizophrenia.

In contrast, Jang, Woodward, Lang, Honer, and Livesley (in press) found no such distinction in a study that estimated the genetic and environmental correlations between the OLIFE and a measure of traits delineating personality disorder on a sample of 102 MZ and 90 DZ general population twin pairs. As noted earlier, schizotypy describes features of personality and psychosis-proneness. Measures of schizotypy like the OLIFE reflect this mix. For this study, the items of the OLIFE were factored to separate personality from psychosis-proneness. Five factors were extracted. Four factors broadly represented personality constructs: extraversion ($h^2_A = 62\%$), nervousness ($h^2_A = 45\%$), lying ($h^2_A = 58\%$), and loneliness or anger ($h^2_A = 58\%$). However, the first and largest factor extracted clearly represented psychotic symptoms and behavior and was called "psychotic features" ($h^2_A = 58\%$).

Substantial genetic correlations were found between the measures of personality disorder traits and all five OLIFE factors. Not surprisingly, the personality disorder trait scales were related to the OLIFE personality factors in predictable ways. For example, the genetic correlation between OLIFE nervousness and anxiousness was .79; the correlation between OLIFE extraversion and social avoidance was .49. Of particular interest is the fact that several personality disorder traits also shared a common genetic basis with OLIFE psychotic features: cognitive distortion ($r_G = .54$), affective lability ($r_G = .55$), stimulus seeking ($r_G = .46$), and suspiciousness ($r_G = .56$). In contrast to the genetic correlations, virtually all of the environmental correlations were small and statistically nonsignificant. These findings highlight the intertwined nature of personality and suggest that schizotypy is a unitary construct and that features from both domains are necessary to properly define the disorder. This relationship is clearly genetically based, but virtually all of the environmental influences on these domains are unique to each, suggesting that the role of the environment is to mediate the differentiation of this genetic liability to either personality or psychosis. This interpretation is consistent with Meehl's (1962) original concept of schizotaxia, in which an inborn neural integrative defect, depending on the type and magnitude of environmental insult, can develop as personality aberrations or schizophrenia when conditions are severe (e.g., childhood trauma).

Steady-State Outcome

Neurodevelopmental models posit that, once developmental processes approach completion, the impact of these alterations in gene expression and their sequelae becomes relatively stabilized. Phenotypically, the symptoms of schizophrenia are stable over time (e.g., Arndt, Andreasen, Flaum, Miller, & Nopoulos, 1995), but the question is whether genetic factors can account for this stability. Does the heritability of schizophrenia change over the lifespan? Do the same genes in early childhood influence the same behaviors in adolescence, adulthood, and old age? These questions are best addressed by classical longitudinal studies of schizophrenic twins. Unfortunately, there have not been any to date. The alternative approach is to perform cross-sectional analyses of twin data from different age groups.

A recent example is Katsanis, Taylor, and Iacono's (2000) study of smooth-pursuit eye-movement dysfunction in preadolescents versus young adults. Smooth-pursuit eye-movement dysfunction is often used as an index of genetic liability in schizophrenia development. Their sample consisted of 64 MZ and 48 DZ twin pairs divided into two age cohorts (11–12 and 17–18 years old). The heritability of both global and specific eye-tracking measures was substantial, accounting for between 40% and 60% of the variance in both groups. The data are consistent with the idea that the same genetic factors are associated with schizophrenia over time. However, the heritability is about half of that observed in adults, suggesting that genetic factors become more salient throughout the lifespan. Clearly, a great deal more work is needed in this area.

SUMMARY

This brief review of some of the behavioral genetic research on schizophrenia provides a solid and consistent evidence for the genetic basis of the disorder. As predicted by this model, the disorder was shown to be consistently and highly heritable across different populations. The lowest is estimate reported is about 70%, and it climbs as high as 85% across schizophrenic phenotypes defined by different diagnostic systems and endophenotypes. The research using endophenotypes is particularly interesting because it suggests that a neural defect is indeed the inherited liability.

Clinical research has identified a number of important environmental traumas, and a growing number of researchers are investigating the mechanisms by which these traumas interact with genetic liabilities to cause—or prevent—development of the disorder. This research, coupled with the theoretical and empirical work on spectrum disorders (e.g., schizotypy and schizoaffective disorder) suggests that what is inherited is a general liability to psychiatric disorder (i.e., schizotaxia), which specific environmental factors can cause to develop into schizophrenia or a personality or a mood disorder. Finally, there appears to be some evidence that the same genetic factors are involved in schizophrenia at different times during the lifespan, but this hypothesis has the least amount of behavioral genetic evidence. The future of behavioral genetic research lies in determining the specific mechanisms, genes, and environmental factors that mediate the development of schizophrenia. Work to date provides broad support for the basic tenets of the neurodevelopmental model, but the devil is in the details.

Chapter 9

Recapitulation

Genes do not fix behavior. Rather, they establish a range of possible reactions to the range of possible experiences that environments can provide.

—Weinberg (1989, p. 101)

It would be reasonable to characterize behavioral genetics research at this time as largely descriptive in nature. Its primary purpose has been to determine what is heritable and to what degree. Over the past two decades the primary research questions has been along the lines of: "Are depression and schizophrenia heritable?," and the answer has been "Yes, about 30% and 80%, respectively." The purpose of multivariate research has been similar. Its task has been to determine why, for example, depressed patients are frequently anxious. The answer has been that depression and anxiety are influenced by some of the same genes.

Finding substantial and significant evidence of heritability for the most common mental disorders bodes well for molecular genetic studies attempting to identify susceptibility loci. These methods promise that, once susceptibility genes are identified, before long it will be possible to screen for psychiatric disorders with blood tests and develop pharmacological interventions to mediate gene function. However, this work has been hampered by the diffuse and heterogeneous nature of many psychiatric phenotypes that may reflect competing genetic and environmental influences. The persistent use of these kinds of broad diagnostic categories is inconsistent with the accumulating evidence from family, adoption, and twin studies that have shown many symptoms defining these categories to be differentially familial or heritable. A key message throughout this book has been that, depending on precisely what is subjected to genetic analysis, quite different answers are found.

The typical approach to overcoming this problem is to design more statistically powerful studies that genotype hundreds or thousands of people worldwide, which allows for the testing of more and more closely spaced alleles. This, coupled with high through-put gene sequencing machines, manages any uncertainty by averaging it out and capitalizing on even minimal true genetic effects through aggregation. The research highlighted in this book, however, suggests that brute force approaches that rely on bigger and faster studies must also be made better by putting greater consideration into the phenotypes subjected to genotyping analysis. The behavioral genetic literature has shown that many of the ways psychopathology is presently understood and conceptualized could do with some revision so that the phenotype accurately reflects its aetiology. Toward this goal, in this short concluding chapter, I briefly summarize the main trends seen in the data and end with some suggestions for critically appraising this research in future.

SUMMARY

The following section enumerates some of the main conclusions that can be drawn from the behavioral genetic literature:

1. Heritability varies according to the disorder. Virtually all disorders have a significant heritable basis. The highest heritabilities have been found with schizophrenia and bipolar depression, at 70% to 80%, with the substance use disorders (e.g., alcoholism) and the personality disorders following at 45% to 55%. The lowest heritabilities are seen with some forms of unipolar depression (around 30%) and the anxiety disorders (20%–45%). Despite the significant genetic basis of the common forms of psychopathology, like a mantra it must be remembered that "heritability does not equal inevitability," because even the most highly heritable disorders can improve with psychological treatment (Gatz, 1990). The work on gene-environment interaction and correlation has demonstrated how genetic and environmental influences mediate the expression of each other. At the level of the individual, genetic factors are thought to impose limits on the degree to which change is possible, and the way to overcome this is to teach people how to adapt to or cope with their conditions (Livesley, 2002, 2003).

2. Many symptoms within any single disorder are differentially heritable. This was not apparent in early heritability studies, which were based on total scores or broad diagnostic categories. Differential heritability of symptoms became clear when studies began to vary the definitions of disorder by including or excluding diagnostic criteria or measuring individual symptoms. An example of the differential heritability of symptoms was demonstrated with social phobia and depression. Not only were symptoms differentially heritable, but within each domain they frequently clustered into aetiologically distinct groups. The important implication of this work is that symptoms could no longer be treated as interchangeable exemplars of a greater syndrome. Rather, each symptom re-

flects the differential influence of common and unique genetic and environmental effects, suggesting that each symptom should be treated as a uniquely inherited entity in its own right and that, given the degree of shared genetic and environmental influence within a group of symptoms, some symptoms are more central as a defining feature of a disorder than others. The implication is that there are some symptoms that should be given more weight in the diagnosis of a disorder, and that this weight can be based in part on the relative influence of genetic and environmental factors. The development of such weights remains a largely unexplored area of research at this time.

3. Environmental effects are largely of the nonshared variety. Heritability analyses have shown that most nonheritable variation in any measured phenotype was accounted for by e^2. In general, c^2 effects have been much smaller. Shared family effects, where they exist, appear to be characteristic of certain disorders. For example, virtually no c^2 effects were found with personality or psychotic disorders, yet they are a consistent feature of the anxiety disorders and of people seeking or undergoing treatment for alcohol abuse and dependence.

It is important to point out here that c^2 effects may have been grossly underestimated because they are confounded with h^2 effects in the typical twins-reared-together design. It has been argued that, unless sample sizes are very large, it is difficult to reliably detect c^2 effects (Neale & Cardon, 1992). The other possibility is that c^2 and even h^2_d effects are present only in specific environmental contexts (e.g., very impoverished or extremely enriched family environments). Estimates of h^2, h^2_d, c^2, and e^2 represent the average across a population and, as such, any effects associated with particular subgroups or environments within a population will be averaged out.

4. Comorbidity is attributable to genetic pleiotropy. Multivariate genetic analyses have shown that the comorbidity between many disorders is attributable to common genetic factors. They also show that environmental factors are largely unique to each disorder. A speculative role of environmental factors is to differentiate disorders, as well as normal and abnormal behavior, or to determine if a general genetic liability to a disorder develops into one of two alternate forms, as suggested by the work on the concept of schizotaxia. The covariance of symptoms within a disorder is also consistent with this pattern.

However, it is not enough to show that variables are related because they share a common genetic basis. It is also important to know how these common genetic and environmental effects are organized, that is, to addresses the question of what, precisely, is inherited. One possibility is that people inherit a general vulnerability to a psychopathology such as major depression. If this is the case, it is possible to treat all symptoms defining a disorder as equal and interchangeable. A diagnosis of major depression can be made using any combination of symptoms, because they all reflect to some degree the influence of a single set of genes. This is the implicit model underlying current present diagnostic systems such as the *DSM*. Behavioral geneticists test the adequacy of this assumption by fitting the common pathways model. The alternative to the common pathways model is the independent pathways model, which states that the coaggregation of symptoms is attributable to a multitude of genetic and environmental factors that directly influence a set of symptoms. In this model, the covariance of the symptoms can be due to several different genetic and environmental factors that influence some but not all of the symptoms. Unlike the common pathways model, syndromes are not inherited. The term *major depression*, for example, is used as a label to describe the covariance of symptoms. Major depression is not inherited, but rather each individual symptom such as moodiness, sleep disturbance, or tearfulness is. They covary because they share some, but not necessarily all, of the same genetic and environmental influences.

In general, contrary to expectation, the common pathways model has not always been found to provide the best explanation for this covariation. Variations of the independent pathways model have often provided a better, or in some cases equally good, fit as the common pathways model. In the latter situation, more theoretical work is required to help provide guidelines for determining which of the two models does indeed reflect the actual structure of symptoms. At the present time, the choice between the equally well-fitting models is largely arbitrary.

5.   Psychopathology is quantitative in nature. The similarity of the magnitude of heritability estimates found between mild and extreme forms of disorder, multivariate analyses of measures of normal and abnormal behavior, and the analysis of general population and clinical samples suggests that disorder exists on a continuum of genetic liability. Several common classes of mental disorder are defined by normal-range behavior at one end (e.g., shyness) and an extreme form at the other (e.g., social phobia) that is caused by unexpressed genes, alternate forms of the same genes, or exposure to a critical environmental event or several events over time. The central idea is that abnormal behavior develops from normal behavior, contrasting with the previous notion that psychopathology develops independently from all other behavior and exists as a stand-alone condition that can be studied and understood without reference to normal behavior. The exception appears to be schizophrenia; this model has not explained the relationship between this disorder and the other functional psychoses. For example, schizophrenia appears to be aetiologically distinct from less severe psychoses (e.g., schizophreniform, schizoaffective, or delusional disorders).

6.   Gene-environment interplay is important. Simply inheriting a liability gene or being exposed to a momentous event often does not lead to mental illness. Genes and the environment influence each other. Two gene-environment interplay effects studied by behavioral geneticists are gene-environment interaction and correlation. Early research had little power to detect these effects, but recent advances in statistical modeling and research design suggest that these effects were previously largely underestimated. There are few studies of these effects currently available, but of those that do exist (e.g., antisocial personality and parental treatment, alcoholism and rural or urban residency), the results are

dramatic. Of particular note is that these new models provide the means to explore environment-by-experience interactions, which to date have received little attention. Just as h^2 can vary over different levels of environmental exposure, so can c^2 and e^2 effects (e.g., attentive mothers mitigating the effects of poverty).

7. Gender-specific factors are important. There is no doubt that some disorders are more prevalent in one gender than another. Sex-limitation analyses have shown that, for many disorders, men and women are influenced by the same genetic and environmental liabilities (e.g., schizophrenia) and only differ in the magnitude of these effects (e.g., anxiety sensitivity and panic). However, there are a number of disorders, such as alcohol abuse, whose variability is attributable to genetic and environmental factors that are largely unique to each gender. Any gender differences in terms of magnitude, genetic effect, or type of effect clearly indicate that gender-specific treatments must not be overlooked.

8. Heritability changes with age. Heritability generally drops with increased age. The same genetic factors appear to be implicated across the lifespan, but their influence on the variability of behavior diminishes. The exception appears to be schizophrenia, whose symptoms remain stable over time; initial evidence suggests that this stability is due in part to genetic influences. In general, there are relatively few longitudinal studies of adult psychopathology and the research on age effects is largely cross-sectional in nature. Most longitudinal behavioral genetic studies at this time focus on infants, children, and young adolescents.

9. Molecular genetic results are mixed. No clear consensus on the location of putative genes or candidates has emerged. There is promising work with endophenotypes and physiological systems beyond the neurotransmitters. These findings also highlight the limitations of current psychiatric diagnostic phenotypes for genetic analyses.

CRITICAL APPRAISAL REVISITED

One purpose of this book was to provide the reader with practical skills in order to digest and critically appraise behavioral genetic research and to appreciate its clinical implications. With this in mind, I reviewed the validity of some early criticisms of the field, including sociopolitical issues and methodological concerns. Basic research designs, statistical methods, and results of published research were discussed in the context of selected issues in psychopathology, such as the validity of the dimensional model or the potential impact of multivariate genetic research on psychiatric classification.

Rutter (2002) discussed at length some new concerns that the field must deal with over the next decade. It is best said in his own words:

> Over the last half century, there has been an explosion of knowledge on the effects of nature, nurture, and developmental processes. As a result, we have a much-improved understanding of many of the mechanisms involved in normal and abnormal development, which carries with it a huge potential for improving

children's lives. Unfortunately, these advances have been accomplished by as much misleading scientific evangelism and journalistic hype as by good science and honest reporting. As a consequence, both the pages of scientific journals and the media have been full of the most absurd confrontations and polarizations. These have given rise to an unhelpful level of misunderstanding of the true scientific advances and, more especially, about their meaning and the implications for policy and practice. Of course, there have also been numerous examples of good reporting by scientists and by journalists. There is every reason to be indebted to both. The need is to avoid the twin dangers of destructive cynicism and gullible expectation. (p. 1)

Behavioral genetic literature has been the victim of misleading presentation of findings, and of extrapolations that have yielded misleading claims that quantitative behavior genetics constitute a causal theory. For example, Rutter (2002) singled out the claim regarding the speed with which susceptibility genes can be found and the extent to which this has clinical utility. Contrary to the claim, none of this will happen very quickly. First, the susceptibility genes must be identified.

This task, reckoned to be the easiest, is already proving to be difficult, despite the mapping of the human genome and some excellent candidates. The search for susceptibility genes is further hampered by a number of methodological issues that the field is only now starting to consider, such as genotype-by-environment interaction. Recent research on cognitive ability suggests that some genes are only expressed in certain environments (Turkheimer, 2003). If susceptibility genes are only expressed in particular environments, then these will first have to be identified and all of the genotyping studies will need to be repeated on individuals and families who were exposed to these environments or are living in them. With respect to research on the environment, Rutter characterized much of it as no more than an attempt to demonstrate a statistical association between some hypothesized risk factor and an outcome variable. Little attention is paid to identifying the actual mechanisms that influence the response to the risk factor. Other issues discussed include geographic and ethnic variability. Presently, it is assumed that susceptibility genes for any particular disorder are a species universal, but this may not be the case.

Even if reliable susceptibility genes are found, Rutter noted that before drug therapies can be developed, scientists have to figure out what the gene actually does. This entails research in three areas: transcriptomics, which ascertains which genes are switched on in particular cells; proteomics, which studies protein interplay within cells; and structural genomics, which studies the dimensional structures of proteins encoded by genes. Rutter's main message for behavioral geneticists is: "To be of any use to policy or practice, it is necessary to know much more with regard to the specifics and how they work" (p. 4).

Behavioral genetics encompasses both genomics and behavioral genomics research. In the not-too-distant future, the distinction will become meaningless, because the study of genetic effects is beginning to affect what is subjected to genotyping analysis, and already many standard twin and adoption methods reviewed in this book have been modified to analyze polymorphisms, to estimate the effects of specific genes and their interplay with environmental factors. Behavioral genetic methods are clearly in a position to provide the means to determine the specifics and how they work. However, the potential of behavioral genetics to provide the why's and the how's will only be realized when behavioral genetic thinking is routinely and fully integrated into all facets of behavioral science research. This is not a difficult task.

Virtually any study conducted by social or behavioral scientists in any discipline can incorporate a new layer of depth by incorporating genetically informative data into the research design. This can be as simple as collecting data on family members (a parent, sibling, or offspring) or collecting data on twins or adoptees. For therapists and other clinicians, behavioral genetic data are vital because they provide evidence (and reassurance to patients and their families) that even the most highly heritable behavior is amenable to change. More importantly, integrating behavioral genetic ideas into clinical thinking will help to determine whether cherished theories and the practices developed from them are based on fortuitous statistical associations or on associations whose basis is intimately tied to our biology and experience.

Further Reading

Behavioral genetics as a field has recently been blessed with a number of books summarizing its vast literature. A few suggested readings are listed here.

Plomin, R., DeFries, J. C., Craig, I. W., & McGuffin, P. (2003). (Eds.). *Behavioral genetics in the postgenomic era*. Washington, DC: American Psychological Association.

The primary focus of this volume is molecular genetic research, but it covers a wide range of topics, including the common psychiatric disorders as well as subjects of interest in mainstream psychology, such as cognitive ability and animal models of emotionality. The book also has an excellent methods section that reviews some of the latest developments in molecular genetic analysis and study design, as well as a chapter that covers factors that hamper the search for susceptibility loci. This book not only reviews previous research, but also explores the future of genetics.

DiLalla, L. F. (Ed.). (2004). *Behavior genetics principles: Perspectives in development, personality, and psychopathology*. Washington, DC: American Psychological Association.

This recently released edited volume provides a broad introduction to a wide variety of topics of interest to psychologists and psychiatrists. The contributors have been drawn from many different backgrounds. Twin, adoption, family, and molecular genetics studies are featured within a developmental context.

McGuffin, P., Owen, M. J., & Gottesman, I. J. (Eds.). (2002). *Psychiatric genetics and genomics*. Oxford: Oxford University Press.

This edited volume provides a very detailed scholarly review of the recent findings in psychiatric genetics. Its primary focus is on molecular genetic research, but it also includes brief reviews of family, twin, and adoption studies. One advantage of this book is that it includes research on a wide range of childhood and adult disorders.

Faraone, S. V., Tsuang, M. T., & Tsuang, D. W. (1999). *Genetics of mental disorders: A guide for students, clinicians, and researchers.* New York: The Guildford Press.

This book provides a good introduction to the methods of psychiatric genetic research. It focuses primarily on molecular genetic research, with detailed examples of its methods. The book discusses clinical implications to some extent, mostly in terms of genetic counseling.

Plomin, R., & McClearn, G. E. (Eds.). (1993). *Nature, nurture and psychology.* Washington, DC: American Psychological Association.

This edited volume reviews the research in several areas of psychology (e.g., personality, cognitive ability, psychopathology, environmental influences, gene-environment interplay), focusing on twin, adoption, and family studies.

References

Almasy, L., Porjesz, B., Blangero, J., Goate, A., Edenberg, H. J., Chorlian, D. B., et al. (2001). Genetics of event-related brain potentials in response to a semantic priming paradigm in families with a history of alcoholism. *American Journal of Human Genetics, 68,* 128–135.

American Psychiatric Association. (1980). *Diagnostic and statistical manual of mental disorders* (3rd ed.). Washington, DC: American Psychiatric Association.

American Psychiatric Association. (1987). *Diagnostic and statistical manual of mental disorders* (3rd ed., rev.). Washington, DC: American Psychiatric Association.

American Psychiatric Association. (1994). *Diagnostic and statistical manual of mental disorders:* (4th ed.). Washington, DC: American Psychiatric Association.

Ando, J., Ono, Y., Yoshimura, K., Onoda, N., Shinohara, M., Kanba, S., et al. (2002). The genetic structure of Cloninger's seven-factor model of temperament and character in a Japanese sample. *Journal of Personality, 70,* 583–610.

Andreasen, N. C. (1983). *The Scale for the Assessment of Negative Symptoms (SANS).* Iowa City: University of Iowa.

Andrews, G., Stewart, G., Allen, R., & Henderson, A.S. (1990). The genetics of six neurotic disorders: A twin study. *Journal of Affective Disorders, 19,* 23–29.

Arndt, S., Andreasen, N. C., Flaum, M., Miller, D., & Nopoulos, P. (1995). A longitudinal study of symptom dimensions in schizophrenia: Prediction and patterns of change. *Archives of General Psychiatry, 52,* 352–360.

Ashton, M. C., Lee, K., Vernon, P. A., & Jang, K. L. (2000). Fluid intelligence, crystallized intelligence, and the Openness/Intellect factor. *Journal of Research in Personality, 3,* 198–207.

Azar, B. (2002). Searching for genes that explain our personalities. *APA Monitor, 33,* 44–46.

Baaré, W. F., van Oel, C. J., Hulshoff, H. E., Schnack, H. G., Durston, S., Sitskoorn, M. M., et al. (2001). Volumes of brain structures in twins discordant for schizophrenia. *Archives of General Psychiatry, 58,* 33–40.

Bailer, U., Leisch, F., Meszaros, K., Lenzinger, E., Willinger, U., Strobl, R., et al. (2000). Genome scan for susceptibility loci for schizophrenia. *Neuropsychobiology, 42,* 175–182.

Bandura, A. (1986). *Social foundations of thought and action: A social cognitive theory.* Rockville, MD: National Institute of Mental Health, Rockville.

Barry, K., & Fleming, M. F. (1990). Family cohesion, expressiveness and conflict in alcoholic families. *British Journal of Addiction, 85,* 81–87.

Battaglia, M., Fossati, A., Torgersen, S., Bertella, S., Bajo, S., Maffei, C., et al. (1999). A psychometric-genetic study of schizotypal disorder. *Schizophrenia Research, 37,* 53–64.

Beck, A. T., & Steer, R. A. (1993). *Beck Depression Inventory manual* (2nd ed.). San Antonio, TX: Harcourt Assessment.

Beckmann, H., Franzek, E., & Stober, G. (1996). Genetic heterogeneity in catatonic schizophrenia: A family study. *American Journal of Medical Genetics, 67,* 289–300.

Begley, S. (2002, June 21). Even thoughts can turn genes on and off. *The Wall Street Journal.*

Benjamin, J., Greenberg, B., & Murphy, D. L. (1996). Mapping personality traits related to genes: Population and family association between the D4 dopamine receptor and measures of novelty seeking. *Nature Genetics, 12,* 81–84.

Bergeman, C. S., Plomin, R., McClearn, G. E., Pedersen, N. L., & Friberg, L. T. (1988). Genotype-environment interaction in personality development: Identical twins reared apart. *Psychology and Aging, 3,* 399–406.

Berman, S. A., Ozkaragoz, T., Young, R. M., & Noble, E. P. (2002). D2 dopamine receptor gene polymorphism discriminates two kinds of novelty seeking. *Personality and Individual Differences, 33,* 867–882.

Bernstein, R. (1971, September). I.Q. *Atlantic Monthly, 229* (1), 43–64.

Berrettini, W. H. (2000). Are schizophrenic and bipolar disorders related? A review of family and molecular studies. *Biological Psychiatry, 48,* 531–538.

Berrettini, W. H., Ferraro, T. N., Goldin, L. R., Weeks, D. E., Detera-Wadleigh, S., Nurnberger, J. I., Jr., et al. (1994). Chromosome 18 DNA markers and manic-depressive illness: Evidence for a susceptibility gene. *Proceedings of the National Academy of Sciences of the United States of America, 91,* 5918–5921.

Bierut, L. J., Dinwiddie, S. H., Begleiter, H., Crowe, R. R., Hesselbrock, V., Nurnberger, J. I., Jr., et al. (1998). Familial transmission of substance dependence: Alcohol, marijuana, cocaine, and habitual smoking: A report from the collaborative study on the genetics of alcoholism. *Archives of General Psychiatry, 55,* 982–988.

Bierut, L. J., Heath, A. C., Bucholz, K. K., Dinwiddie, S. H., Madden, P. A., Statham, D. J., et al. (1999). Major depressive disorder in a community-based twin sample: Are there different genetic and environmental contributions for men and women? *Archives of General Psychiatry, 56,* 557–563.

Black, D. W., Goldstein, R. B., Noyes, R., Jr., & Blum, N. (1995). Psychiatric disorders in relatives of probands with obsessive-compulsive disorder and co-morbid major depression or generalized anxiety. *Psychiatric Genetics, 5,* 37–41.

Blehar, M. C., & Lewy, A. J. (1990). Seasonal mood disorders: Consensus and controversy. *Psychopharmacology Bulletin, 26,* 465–494.

Bleuler, E. (1950). *Dementia praecox: Or, the group of schizophrenias* (J. Zinkin, trans.), New York : International Universities Press.

Blouin, J. L., Dombroski, B. A., Nath, S. K., Lasseter, V. K., Wolyniec, P. S., Nestadt, G., et al. (1998). Schizophrenia susceptibility loci on chromosomes 13q32 and 8p21. *Nature Genetics, 20,* 70–73.

Blum, K., Noble, E. P., Sheridan, P. J., Montgomery, A., Ritchie, T., Jagadeeswaran, P., et al. (1990). Allelic association of human dopamine-D2 receptor gene in alcoholism. *JAMA, 263,* 2055–2060.

Bolos, A. M., Dean, M., Lucas-Derse, S., Ramsburg, M., Brown, G. L., Goldman, D. (1990). Population and pedigree studies reveal a lack of association between the dopamine D2 receptor gene and alcoholism. *JAMA, 264*, 3156–3160.

Boomsma, D. I. (1996). Using multivariate genetic modeling to detect pleiotropic quantitative trait loci. *Behavior Genetics, 26*, 161–166.

Borkenau, P., Riemann, R., Angleitner, A., & Spinath, F. M. (2002). Similarity of childhood experiences and personality resemblance in monozygotic and dizygotic twins: A test of the equal environments assumption. *Personality and Individual Differences, 33*, 261–269.

Bouchard, T. J., Jr. (1997). The genetics of personality. In K. Blum, & E. P. Noble (Eds.), *Handbook of psychiatric genetics* (pp. 273–296). Boca Raton, FL: CRC Press.

Bouchard, T. J., Jr., & Loehlin, J. C. (2001). Genes, evolution, and personality. *Behavior Genetics, 31*, 243–273.

Bouwer, C., & Stein, D. J. (1997). Association of panic disorder with a history of traumatic suffocation. *American Journal of Psychiatry, 154*, 1566–1570.

Boyce, P., & Parker, G. (1988). Seasonal affective disorder in the southern hemisphere. *Journal of Psychiatry, 145*, 96–99.

Breslau, N., Davis, G. C., Andreski, P., & Peterson, E. (1991). Traumatic events and posttraumatic stress disorder in an urban population of young adults. *Archives of General Psychiatry, 48*, 216–222.

Brown, G. W., Harris, T. O., Hepworth, C., & Robinson, R. (1994). Clinical and psychosocial origins of chronic depressive episodes: Vol. 2. A patient enquiry. *British Journal of Psychiatry, 165*, 457–465.

Brown, G. W., Harris, T. O., & Hepworth, C. (1994). Life events and endogenous depression: A puzzle reexamined. *Archives of General Psychiatry, 51*, 525–534.

Brown, G. W. (1998).Genetic and population perspectives on life events and depression. *Social Psychiatry and Psychiatric Epidemiology, 33*, 363–372.

Burt, S. A., McGue, M., Iacono, W., Comings, D., & MacMurray, J. (2002). An examination of the association between DRD4 and DRD2 polymorphisms and personality traits. *Personality and Individual Differences, 33*, 849–860.

Byerley, W., Hoff, M., Holik, J., & Coon, H. (1994). A linkage study with D5 dopamine and 1a-sub(2c)-adrenergic receptor genes in six multiplex bipolar pedigrees. *Psychiatric Genetics, 4*, 121–124.

Cadoret, R. J., Yates, W. R., Troughton, E., Woodworth, G. W., & Stewart, M. A. (1995). Adoption study demonstrating two genetic pathways to drug abuse. *Archives of General Psychiatry, 52*, 42–52.

Cadoret, R. J., Winokur, G., Langbehn, D., & Troughton, E. (1996). Depression spectrum disease I: The role of gene-environment interaction. *American Journal of Psychiatry, 153*, 892–899.

Cannon, T. D., Kaprio, J., Loennquist, J., Huttunen, M., & Koskenvuo, M. (1998). The genetic epidemiology of schizophrenia in a Finnish twin cohort: A population-based modeling study. *Archives of General Psychiatry, 55*, 67–74.

Cardno, A. G., Marshall, E. J., Coid, B., Macdonald, A. M., Ribchester, T. R., Davies, N. J., et al. (1999). Heritability estimates for psychotic disorders: The Maudsley twin psychosis series. *Archives of General Psychiatry, 56*, 162–168.

Cardno, A. G., Sham, P. C., Farmer, A. E., Murray, R. M., & McGuffin, P. (2002). Heritability of Schneider's first-rank symptoms. *British Journal of Psychiatry, 180*, 35–38.

Cardon, L. R., Smith, S. D., Fulker, D. W., Kimberling, W. J., Pennington, B. F., & DeFries, J. C. (1994, October). Quantitative trait locus for reading disability on chromosome 6. *Science, 266*, 276–279.

Carey, G., & DiLalla, D. L. (1994). Personality and psychopathology: Genetic perspectives. *Journal of Abnormal Psychology, 103*, 32–43.

Caspi, A., McClay, J., & Moffitt, T. (2002, August). Role of genotype in the cycle of violence in maltreated children. *Science, 297*, 851–854.

Chaldee, M., Corbex, M., Campion, D., Jay, M., Samolyk, D., Petit, M., et al. (2001). No evidence for linkage between COMT and schizophrenia in a French population. *Psychiatry Research, 102*, 87–90.

Chambless, D. L., & Gracely, E. J. (1988). Predictors of outcome following in vivo exposure treatment of agoraphobia. In I. Hand, H. U. Wittchen (Eds.), *Panic and phobias II: Treatment and variables affecting outcome.* New York: Springer-Verlag.

Charney, D. S., Barlow, D. H., & Botteron, K. (2002). Neuroscience research agenda to guide development of a pathophysiologically based classification system. *In A Research Agenda For DSM-V,* Kupfer, D. J., First, M. B., Rieger, D. A. (Eds). Washington DC: American Psychiatric Association, 2002.

Cherny, S. S., DeFries, J. C., & Fulker, D. W. (1992). Multiple regression analysis of twin data: A model-fitting approach. *Behavior Genetics, 22*, 489–497.

Clark, D. M., & Wells, A. (1997). Cognitive therapy for anxiety disorders. In L. J. Dickstein, M. B. Riba (Eds.), *American Psychiatric Press review of psychiatry* (Vol. 16, pp, 19–143). Washington: American Psychiatric Press.

Cloninger, C. R. (1986). A unified biosocial theory of personality and its role in the development of anxiety states. *Psychiatric Developments, 3*, 167–226.

Cloninger, C. R. (1994). Temperament and personality. *Current Opinion in Neurobiology, 4*, 266–273.

Cloninger, C. R., Adolfsson, R., & Svrakic, N. M. (1996). Mapping genes for human personality. *Nature Genetics, 12*, 3–4.

Cloninger, C. R., Przybeck, T., Svrakic, D., & Wetzel, R. D. (1994). *The Temperament and Character Inventory (TCI): A guide to its development and use.* St. Louis, MO: Washington University. Center for Psychobiology and Personality.

Cloninger, C. R., Svrakic, D. M., & Przybeck, T. R. (1993). A psychobiological model of temperament and character. *Archives of General Psychiatry, 50*, 975–990.

Collier, D. A., Arranz, M. J., Sham, P., & Battersby, S. (1996). The serotonin transporter is a potential susceptibility factor for bipolar affective disorder. *Neuroreport, 7,* 1675–1679.

Conrod, P. J., Peterson, J. B., & Pihl, R. O. (2001). Reliability and validity of alcohol-induced heart rate increase as a measure of sensitivity to the stimulant properties of alcohol. *Psychopharmacology, 157,* 20–30.

Costa, P. T., & McCrae, R. R. (1992). *Revised NEO Personality Inventory and NEO Five-Factor Inventory.* Odessa, FL: Psychological Assessment Resources.

Costa, P. T., & Widiger, T. A., (Eds.). (1994). *Personality disorders and the five-factor model of personality.* Washington, DC: American Psychological Association.

Cowen, P. J. (1993). Serotonin receptor subtypes in depression: Evidence from studies in neuroendocrine regulation. *Clinical Neuropharmacology, 16*(Suppl. 3), S6–S18.

Crawford, C. B. (1979). George Washington, Abraham Lincoln and Arthur Jensen: Are they compatible? *American Psychologist, 34*, 664–672.

Dahl, A. A. (1993). The personality disorders: A critical review of family, twin, and adoption studies. *Journal of Personality Disorders Vol.7* (Suppl. 1), 86–99.

Dalman, C., Allebeck, P., Cullberg, J., Grunewald, C., & Koster, M. (1999). Obstetric complications and the risk of schizophrenia: A longitudinal study of a national birth cohort. *Archives of General Psychiatry, 56*, 234–240.

DeFries, J. C., & Fulker, D. W. (1985). Multiple regression analysis of twin data. *Behavior Genetics, 15*, 467–473.

DeFries, J. C., & Fulker, D. W. (1988). Multiple regression analysis of twin data: Etiology of deviant scores versus individual differences. *Acta Geneticae Medicae et Gemellologiae: Twin Research, 37*, 205–216.

De Fruyt, F., Van De Wiele, L., & Van Heeringen, C. (2000). Cloninger's psychobiological model of temperament and character and the five-factor model of personality. *Personality and Individual Differences, 29*, 441–452.

Depue, R. A., & Collins, P. F. (1999). Neurobiology of the structure of personality: Dopamine, facilitation of incentive motivation, and extraversion. *Behavioral and Brain Sciences, 22*, 491–569.

Derogatis, L. R. (1994). *Symptom Checklist-90-R administration, scoring, and procedures manual* (3rd ed.). Minneapolis, MN: National Computer Systems.

Detera-Wadleigh, S. D., Badner, J. A., Berrettini, W. H., Yoshikawa, T. Goldin, L. R., Turner, G., et al. (1999). A high-density genome scan detects evidence for a bipolar-disorder susceptibility locus on 13q32 and other potential loci on 1q32 and 18p11.2. *Proceedings of the National Academy of Sciences of the United States of America, 96*, 5604–5609.

Dick, D. M., Rose, R. J., Viken, R. J., Kaprio, J., & Koskenvuo, M. (2001). Exploring gene-environment interactions: Socioregional moderation of alcohol use. *Journal of Abnormal Psychology, 110*, 625–632.

DiLalla, D. L., Carey, G., Gottesman, I. I., & Bouchard, T. J., Jr. (1996). Heritability of MMPI personality indicators of psychopathology in twins reared apart. *Journal of Abnormal Psychology, 105*, 491–499.

Dunn, G., Sham, P. C., & Hand, D. (1993). Statistics and the nature of depression. *Psychological Medicine, 23*, 871–889.

Eaves, L. J., Eysenck, H. J., & Martin, N. G. (1989). *Genes, culture and personality: An empirical approach*. London: Oxford University Press.

Eaves, L. J., & Meyer, J. (1994). Locating human quantitative trait loci: Guidelines for the selection of sibling pairs for genotyping. *Behavior Genetics, 24*, 443–455.

Ebstein, R. P., Novick, O., & Umansky, R. (1996). D4DR exon III polymorphism associated with the personality trait of novelty seeking in normal human volunteers. *Nature Genetics, 12*, 78–80.

Ebstein, R. P., Gritsenko, I., & Nemanov, L. (1997). No association between the serotonin transporter gene regulatory region polymorphism and the tridimensional personality questionnaire (TPQ) temperament of harm avoidance. *Molecular Psychiatry, 2*, 224–226.

Ebstein, R. P., Segman, R., & Benjamin, J. (1997). 5-HT2C (HTR2C) serotonin receptor gene polymorphism associated with the human personality trait of reward dependence: Interaction with dopamine D4 receptor (D4DR) and dopamine D3 (D3DR) polymorphisms. *American Journal of Medical Genetics, 74*, 65–72.

Eysenck, H. J., & Eysenck, S. B. G. (1992). *Manual for the Eysenck Personality Questionnaire* (rev. ed.). San Diego, CA: Educational and Industrial Testing Service.

Fagerstrom, K. O., & Schneider, N. G. (1989). Measuring nicotine dependence: A review of the Fagerstrom Tolerance Questionnaire. *Journal of Behavioral Medicine, 12*, 159–182.

Falconer, D. S. (1960). *Introduction to quantitative genetics*. New York: Ronald Press.

Fauerbach, J. A., Lawrence, J. W., & Schmidt, C. W., Jr. (2000). Personality predictors of injury-related posttraumatic stress disorder. *Journal of Nervous and Mental Disease, 188*, 510–517.

Feighner, J. P., Robins, E., & Guze, S. B. (1972). Diagnostic criteria for use in psychiatric research. *Archives of General Psychiatry, 26*, 57–63.

Feinstein, A. R. (1970). The pretherapeutic classification of co-morbidity in chronic disease. *Journal of Chronic Disorders, 23*, 455–468.

Finkel, D., & McGue, M. (1997). Sex differences and nonadditivity in heritability of the Multidimensional Personality Questionnaire scales. *Journal of Personality and Social Psychology, 72*, 929–938.

Franzek, E., & Beckmann, H. (1998). Different genetic background of schizophrenia spectrum psychosis: A twin study. *American Journal of Psychiatry, 155*, 76–83.

Garmezy, N., & Masten, A. S. (1994). Chronic adversities. In M. Rutter & L. Hersov (Eds.), *Child and adolescent psychiatry: Modern approaches* (3rd ed., pp. 191–208). London: Blackwell.

Gatz, M. (1990). Interpreting behavior genetic results: Suggestions for counselors and clients. *Journal of Counseling and Development, 68,* 601–605.

Gebhardt, C., Fureder, T., Fuchs, K., Urmann, A., Gerhard, E., Heiden, A., et al. (1997, October). *No evidence for normal personality traits related to dopamine 4 receptor gene polymorphism.* Paper presented at the 1997 World Congress on Psychiatric Genetics, Santa Fe, NM.

Geijer, T., Frisch, A., Persson, M. L., Wasserman, D., Rockah, R., Michaelovsky, E., et al. (2000). Search for associations between suicide attempt and serotonergic polymorphisms. *Psychiatric Genetics, 10,* 19–26.

Gelernter, J., Kranzler, H., Coccaro, E. F., Siever, L. J., & New, A. S. (1998). Serotonin transporter protein gene polymorphism and personality measures in African American and European American subjects. *American Journal of Psychiatry, 155,* 1332–1338.

Gershon, E. S., Badner, J. A., Goldin, L. R., Sanders, A. R., Cravchik, A., & Detera-Wadleigh, S. D. (1998). Closing in on genes for manic-depressive illness and schizophrenia. *Neuropsychopharmacology, 18,* 233–242.

Gershon, E. S. (2000). Bipolar illness and schizophrenia as oligogenic diseases: Implications for the future. *Biological Psychiatry, 47,* 240–244.

Gottesman, I. I. (1991). *Schizophrenia genesis: The origins of madness.* New York: Freeman.

Gough, H. G. (1989). The California Psychological Inventory. In C. S. Newmark (Ed.), *Major psychological assessment instruments* (Vol. 2, pp. 67–98). Needham Heights, MA: Allyn and Bacon.

Grant, B. F., & Dawson, D. A. (1997). Age at onset of alcohol use and its association with *DSM-IV* alcohol abuse and dependence: Results from the National longitudinal alcohol epidemiologic survey. *Journal of Substance Abuse, 9,* 103–110.

Greene, R. L. (1991). *The MMPI-2/MMPI: An interpretive manual.* Boston, MA: Allyn and Bacon.

Hafner, J. R. (1983). Behaviour therapy for agoraphobic men. *Behavior, Research, and Therapy, 21,* 51–56.

Grove, W. M., Eckert, E. D., Heston, L., Bouchard, T. J., Jr., Segal, N., & Lykken, D. (1990). Heritability of substance abuse and antisocial behavior: A study of monozygotic twins reared apart. *Biological Psychiatry, 27,* 1293–1304.

Hamer, D. H., & Copeland, P. (1998). *Living with our genes: Why they matter more than you think.* New York: Doubleday.

Hamer, D. H., Greenberg, B. D., Sabol, S. Z., & Murphy, D. L. (1999). Role of serotonin transporter gene in temperament and character. *Journal of Personality Disorders, 13,* 312–328.

Hamilton, M. (1967). Development of a rating scale for primary depressive illness. *British Journal of Social and Clinical Psychology, 6,* 278–96.

Hamilton, S. P., Haghighi, F., Heiman, G. A., Klein, D. F., Hodge, S. E., Fyer, A. J., et al. (2000). Investigation of dopamine receptor (DRD4) and dopamine transporter (DAT) polymorphisms for genetic linkage or association to panic disorder. *American Journal of Medical Genetics, 96,* 324–330.

Hamilton, S. P., Heiman, G. A., Haghighi, F., Mick, S., Klein, D. F., Hodge, S. E., et al. (1999). Lack of genetic linkage or association between a functional serotonin transporter polymorphism and panic disorder. *Psychiatric Genetics, 9,* 1–6.

Han, C., McGue, M. K., & Iacono, W. G. (1999). Lifetime tobacco, alcohol and other substance use in adolescent Minnesota twins: Univariate and multivariate behavioral genetic analyses. *Addiction, 94,* 981–993.

Harris, J. R. (1998). *The nurture assumption.* New York: Simon and Schuster.

Hariri, A. R., Mattay, V. S., & Tessitore, A. (2002, July). Serotonin transporter genetic variation and the response of the human amygdala. *Science, 297,* 400–403.

Harvey, J. M., & Dodd, D. K. (1995). Children of alcoholics, negative life events, and early experimentation with drugs. *Journal of School Psychology, 33,* 305–317.

Heath, A. C., Bucholz, K. K., & Slutske, W. S. (1994). The assessment of alcoholism in surveys of the general community: What are we measuring? Some insights from the Australian twin panel interview survey. *International Review of Psychiatry, 6,* 295–307.

Heath, A. C., Bucholz, K. K., Madden, P. A. F., Dinwiddie, S. H., Slutske, W. S., Bierut, L. J., et al. (1997). Genetic and environmental contributions to alcohol dependence risk in a national twin sample: Consistency of findings in women and men. *Psychological Medicine, 27,* 1381–1396.

Heath, A. C., Eaves, L. J., & Martin, N. G. (1989). The genetic structure of personality: III. Multivariate genetic item analysis of the EPQ scales. *Personality and Individual Differences, 10,* 877–888.

Heath, A. C., Madden, P. A. F., Grant, J. D., McLaughlin, T. L., Todorov, A. A., & Bucholz, K. K. (1999). Resiliency factors protecting against teenage alcohol use and smoking: Influences of religion, religious involvement and values, and ethnicity in the Missouri Adolescent Female Twin Study. *Twin Research, 2,* 145–155.

Heath, A. C., Martin, N. G., Lynskey, M. T., Todorov, A. A., Madden, P. A. (2002). Estimating two-stage models for genetic influences on alcohol, tobacco or drug use initiation and dependence vulnerability in twin and family data. *Twin Research, 5,* 113–124.

Helmuth, L. (2003, October 31). In sickness or in health? *Science, 303,* 808–810.

Hesselbrock ,V., Begleiter, H., Porjesz, B., O'Connor, S., & Bauer, L. (2001). P300 event-related potential amplitude as an endophenotype of alcoholism: Evidence from the collaborative study on the genetics of alcoholism. *Journal of Biomedical Science, 8,* 77–82.

Hettema, J. M., Neale, M. C., & Kendler, K. S. (2001). A review and meta-analysis of the genetic epidemiology of anxiety disorders. *American Journal of Psychiatry, 158,* 1568–1578.

Hettema, J. M., Prescott, C. A., & Kendler, K. S. (2001). A population-based twin study of generalized anxiety disorder in men and women. *Journal of Nervous and Mental Disease, 189,* 413–420.

Hettema, J. M., Annas, P., & Neale, M. C. (2003). A twin study of the genetics of fear conditioning. *Archives of General Psychiatry, 60,* 702–708.

Holmes, D. S., Brynjolfsson, J., Brett, P., & Curtis, D. (1991). No evidence for a susceptibility locus predisposing to manic depression in the region of the dopamine (D2) receptor gene. *British Journal of Psychiatry, 158,* 635–641.

Holmes, S. J., & Robins, L. N. (1988). The role of parental disciplinary practices in the development of depression and alcoholism. *Psychiatry: Journal for the Study of Interpersonal Processes, 51,* 24–36.

Jang, K. L., Lam, R. W., Livesley, W. J., & Vernon, P. A. (1997). The relationship between seasonal mood change and personality: More apparent than real? *Acta Psychiatrica Scandinavica, 95,* 539–543.

Jang, K. L., Livesley, W. J., & Vernon, P. A. (1995). Alcohol and drug problems: A multivariate behavioural genetic analysis of comorbidity. *Addiction, 90,* 1213–1221.

Jang, K. L., Livesley, W. J., & Vernon, P. A. (1996). Heritability of the Big Five personality dimensions and their facets: A twin study. *Journal of Personality, 64,* 577–591.

Jang, K. L., Livesley, W. J., Vernon, P. A. (1998). A twin study of genetic and environmental contributions to gender differences in traits delineating personality disorder. *European Journal of Personality, 12,* 331–344.

Jang, K. L., & Livesley, W. J. (1999). Why do measures of normal and disordered personality correlate? A study of genetic comorbidity. *Journal of Personality Disorders, 13,* 10–17.

Jang, K. L., McCrae, R. R., Angleitner, A., Riemann, R., & Livesley, W. J. (1998). Heritability of facet-level traits in a cross-cultural twin sample: Support for a hierarchical model of personality. *Journal of Personality and Social Psychology, 74,* 1556–1565.

Jang, K. L., Stein, M. B., Taylor, S., & Livesley, W. J. (1999). Gender differences in the etiology of anxiety sensitivity: A twin study. *Journal of Gender-Specific Medicine, 2,* 39–44.

Jang, K. L., Livesley, W. J., Angleitner, A., Riemann, R., & Vernon, P. A. (2002). Genetic and environmental influences on the covariance of facets defining the domains of the Five-Factor Model of personality. *Personality and Individual Differences, 33,* 83–101.

Jang, K. L., Vernon, P. A., & Livesley, W. J. (2000). Personality disorder traits, family environment, and alcohol misuse: A multivariate behavioural genetic analysis. *Addiction, 95,* 873–888.

Jang, K. L., Vernon, P. A., Livesley, W. J., Stein, M. B., & Wolf, H. (2001). Intra-and extra-familial influences on alcohol and drug misuse: A twin study of genetic-environmental correlations. *Addiction, 96,* 1307–1318.

Jang, K. L., Stein, M. B., Taylor, S., Asmundson, G., & Livesley, W. J. (2003). Exposure to traumatic events and experience: Aetiological relationships with personality function. *Psychiatry Research, 120,* 61–69.

Jang, K. L., Livesley, W. J., Vernon, P. A., Taylor, S., & Moon, E. C. (2004). Heritability of individual depressive symptoms. *Journal of Affective Disorders, 80,* 125–133.

Jang, K. L., Woodward, T. S., Lang, D., Honer, W. G., & Livesley, W. J. (in press). The genetic and environmental basis of the relationship between schizotypy and personality: A twin study. *Journal of Nervous and Mental Disease.*

Jansen, M. A., Arntz, A., Merckelbach, H., & Mersch, P. P. A. (1994). Personality disorders and features in social phobia and panic disorder. *Journal of Abnormal Psychology, 103,* 391–395.

Jensen, A. R. (1969). How much can we boost IQ and scholastic achievement? *Harvard Educational Review, 39,* 1–123.

Johansson, C., Smedh, C., Partonen, T., Pekkarinen, P., Paunio, T., Ekholm, J., et al. (2001). Seasonal affective disorder and serotonin-related polymorphisms. *Neurobiology of Disease, 8,* 351–357.

Johnson, W., & Krueger, R. F. (in press). Genetic and environmental structure of adjectives describing the domains of the Big Five Model of Personality: A nationwide US twin study. *Journal of Abnormal Psychology.*

Jonnal, A. H., Gardner, C. O., Prescott, C. A., & Kendler, K. S. (2000). Obsessive and compulsive symptoms in a general population sample of female twins. *American Journal of Medical Genetics, 96,* 791–796.

Kamin, L. J. (1974). *The science and politics of IQ.* New York: Halsted.

Kamin, L. J. & Goldberger, A. S. (2002). Twin studies in behavioral research: A skeptical view. *Theoretical Population Biology, 61,* 83–95.

Kasriel, J., & Eaves, L. J. (1976). The zygosity of twins: Further evidence on the agreement between diagnosis by blood groups and written questionnaires. *Journal of Biosocial Science, 8,* 263–266.

Katsanis, J., Taylor, J., & Iacono, W. G. (2000). Heritability of different measures of smooth pursuit eye tracking dysfunction: A study of normal twins. *Psychophysiology, 37,* 724–730.

Katsuragi, S., Kunugi, H., Sano, A., Tsutsumi, T., Isogawa, K., Nanko, S., et al. (1999). Association between serotonin transporter gene polymorphism and anxiety related traits. *Biological Psychiatry, 45,* 368–370.

Kendler, K. S. (1985). Diagnostic approaches to schizotypal personality disorder: A historical perspective. *Schizophrenia Bulletin, 11,* 538–553.

Kendler, K. S., & Eaves, L. J. (1986). Models for the joint effect of genotype and environment on liability to psychiatric illness. *American Journal of Psychiatry, 143,* 279–289.

Kendler, K. S., Heath, A. C., Neale, M. C., Kessler, R. C., & Eaves, L. J. (1992). A population-based twin study of alcoholism in women. *JAMA, 268*, 1877–1882.

Kendler, K. S., Karkowski, L. M., & Walsh, D. (1998). The structure of psychosis: Latent class analysis of probands from the Roscommon Family Study. *Archives of General Psychiatry, 55*, 492–499.

Kendler, K. S., Karkowski, L. M., & Prescott, C. A. (1999). The assessment of dependence in the study of stressful life events: Validation using a twin design. *Psychological Medicine, 29*, 1455–1460.

Kendler, K. S., Karkowski, L. M., Corey, L. A., Prescott, C. A., & Neale, M. C. (1999). Genetic and environmental risk factors in the aetiology of illicit drug initiation and subsequent misuse in women. *British Journal of Psychiatry, 175*, 351–356.

Kendler, K. S., & Karkowski-Shuman, L. (1997). Stressful life events and genetic liability to major depression: Genetic control of exposure to the environment? *Psychological Medicine, 27*, 539–547.

Kendler, K. S., Lieberman, J. A., & Walsh, D. (1989). The Structured Interview for Schizotypy (SIS): A preliminary report. *Schizophrenia Bulletin, 15*, 559–571.

Kendler, K. S., Kessler, R. C., Walters, E. E., MacLean, C., Neale, M. C. Heath, A. C., et al. (1995). Stressful life events, genetic liability, and onset of an episode of major depression in women. *American Journal of Psychiatry, 152*, 833–842.

Kendler, K. S., Neale, M. C., Kessler, R. C., Heath, A., & Eaves, L. J. (1992a). A population-based twin study of major depression in women. *Archives of General Psychiatry, 49*, 257–266.

Kendler, K. S., Neale, M. C., Kessler, R. C., Heath, A.C., & Eaves, L. J. (1992b). Generalized anxiety disorder in women: A population-based twin study. *Archives of General Psychiatry, 49*, 267–272.

Kendler, K. S., Neale, M. C., Kessler, R. C., Heath, A., & Eaves, L. J. (1992c). Major depression and generalized anxiety disorder: Same genes, (partly) different environments? *Archives of General Psychiatry, 49*, 716–722.

Kendler, K. S., Neale, M. C., Kessler, R. C., Heath, A. C. & Eaves, L. J. (1992d) The genetic epidemiology of phobias in women: The interrelationship of agoraphobia, social phobia, situational phobia, and simple phobia. *Archives of General Psychiatry, 49*, 273–281.

Kendler, K. S., Neale, M. C., Kessler, R. C., Heath, A. C., & Eaves, L. J. (1993). The lifetime history of major depression in women: Reliability of diagnosis and heritability. *Archives of General Psychiatry, 50*, 863–870.

Kendler, K. S., Neale, M. C., Kessler, R. C., Heath A. C., & Eaves, L. J.(1993). Panic disorder in women: A population-based twin study. *Psychological Medicine, 23*, 397–406.

Kendler, K. S., Neale, M. C., Kessler, R. C., & Heath, A. C. (1994). Parental treatment and the equal environment assumption in twin studies of psychiatric illness. *Psychological Medicine, 24*, 579–590.

Kendler, K. S., Pedersen, N. L., Neale, M. C., & Mathé, A. A. (1995). A pilot Swedish twin study of affective illness including hospital- and population-ascertained subsamples: Results of model fitting. *Behavior Genetics, 25*, 217–232.

Kendler, K. S., Neale, M. C., Sullivan, P., Corey, L. A., Gardner, C. O., & Prescott, C. A. (1999). A population-based twin study in women of smoking initiation and nicotine dependence. *Psychological Medicine, 29*, 299–308.

Kendler, K. S., & Prescott, C. A. (1999a). A population-based twin study of lifetime major depression in men and women. *Archives of General Psychiatry, 5*, 39–44.

Kendler, K. S., & Prescott, C. A. (1999b). Caffeine intake, tolerance, and withdrawal in women: A population-based twin study. *American Journal of Psychiatry, 156*, 223–228.

Kendler, K. S., Thornton, L. M., & Gardner, C. O. (2000). Stressful life events and previous episodes in the etiology of major depression in women: An evaluation of the "kindling" hypothesis. *American Journal of Psychiatry, 157,* 1243–1251.

Kendler, K. S., Walters, E. E., Neale, M. C., Kessler, R. C., Heath, A. C., & Eaves, L. J. (1995). The structure of the genetic and environmental risk factors for six major psychiatric disorders in women: Phobia, generalized anxiety disorder, panic disorder, bulimia, major depression, and alcoholism. *Archives of General Psychiatry, 52,* 374–383.

Kendler, K. S., Walters, E. E., Truett, K. R., Heath, A. C., Neale, M. C., Martin, N. G., et al. (1995). A twin-family study of self-report symptoms of panic-phobia and somatization. *Behavior Genetics, 25,* 499–515.

Kendler, K. S., Myers, J., & Prescott, C. A. (2002). The etiology of phobias: An evaluation of the stress-diathesis model. *Archives of General Psychiatry, 59,* 242–248.

Kendler, K. S., Prescott, C. A., Myers, J., & Neale, M. C. (2003). The structure of genetic and environmental risk factors for common psychiatric and substance use disorders in men and women. *Archives of General Psychiatry, 60,* 929–937.

Kessler, R. C., McGonagle, K. A.,& Zhao, S. (1994). Lifetime and 12-month prevalence of DSM-III-R psychiatric disorders in the United States. *Archives of General Psychiatry, 51,* 8–19.

Kilpatrick, D. G., Resnick, H. S., Saunders, B. E., & Best, C. L. (1998). Rape, other violence against women, and posttraumatic stress disorder. In B. P. Dohrenwend, (Ed.), *Adversity, stress, and psychopathology* (pp. 161–176). London: Oxford University Press.

King, J. A., Abend, S., & Edwards, E. (2001). Genetic predisposition and the development of posttraumatic stress disorder in an animal model. *Biological Psychiatry, 50,* 231–237.

King, D. W., King, L. A., Foy, D. W., Keane, T. M., & Fairbank, J. A. (1999). Posttraumatic stress disorder in a national sample of female and male Vietnam veterans: Risk factors, war-zone stressors, and resilience-recovery variables. *Journal of Abnormal Psychology, 108,* 164–170.

Kitao, Y., Inada, T., Arinami, T., Hirotsu, C., Aoki, S., Iijima, Y., et al. (2000). A contribution to genome-wide association studies: Search for susceptibility loci for schizophrenia using DNA microsatellite markers on chromosome 19, 20, 21 and 22. *Psychiatric Genetics, 10,* 139–143.

Knutson, B., Wolkowitz, O. M., Cole, S. W., Chan, T., Moore, E. A., Johnson, R. C., et al. (1998). Selective alteration of personality and social behavior by serotonergic intervention. *American Journal of Psychiatry, 155,* 373–379.

Koenen, K. C., Harley, R., Lyons, M. J., Wolfe, J., Simpson, J. C., Goldberg, J., et al. (2002). A twin registry study of familial and individual risk factors for trauma exposure and posttraumatic stress disorder. *Journal of Nervous and Mental Disease. 190,* 209–218.

Koopmans, J. R., Slutske, W. S., Van Baal, C. M., & Boomsma, D. I. (1999). The influence of religion on alcohol use initiation: Evidence for a genotype environment interaction. *Behavior Genetics, 29,* 445–453.

Kraepelin, E. (1919). *Of dementia præcox and paraphrenia* (R. M. Barclay, Trans.). G. M. Robertson (Ed.), Textbook of psychiatry (8th Ed). Edinburgh, Scotland: Livingstone.

Krueger, R. F. (1999). The structure of common mental disorders. *Archives of General Psychiatry, 56,* 921–926.

Krueger, R. F., McGue, M., & Iacono, W. G. (2001). The higher-order structure of common *DSM* mental disorders: Internalization, externalization, and their connections to personality. *Personality and Individual Differences, 30,* 1245–1259.

Krueger, R. F., Hicks, B. M., Patrick, C. J., Carlson, S. R., Iacono, W. G., & McGue, M. (2002). Etiologic connections among substance dependence, antisocial behavior, and personality: Modeling the externalizing spectrum. *Journal of Abnormal Psychology, 111,* 411–424.

Kurumaji, A., Nomoto, H., Yamada, K., Yoshikawa, T., & Toru, M. (2001). No association of two missense variations of the benzodiazepine receptor (peripheral) gene and mood disorders in a Japanese sample. *American Journal of Medical Genetics, 105,* 172–175.

Lachman, H. M., Papolos, D. F., Saito, T., Yu, Y. M., Szumlanski, C. L., & Weinshilboum, R. M. (1996). Human catechol-O-methyltransferase pharmacogenetics: Description of a functional polymorphism and its potential application to neuropsychiatric disorders. *Pharmacogenetics, 6*, 243–250.

Lam, R. W., Kripke, D. F., & Gillin, J. C. (1989). Phototherapy for depressive disorders: A review. *Canadian Journal of Psychiatry-Revue Canadienne de Psychiatrie, 34*, 140–147.

Lander, E. S., & Botstein, D. (1989). Mapping mendalian factors underlying quantitative traits using RFLP linkage maps. *Genetics, 121*, 185–199.

Larstone, R. M., Jang, K. L., Livesley, W. J., Vernon, P. A., & Wolf, H. (2002). The relationship between Eysenck's P-E-N model of personality, the five-factor model of personality, and traits delineating personality disorder. *Personality and Individual Differences, 33*, 25–37.

Leary, M. R., & Kowalski, R. M. (1995).The self-presentation model of social phobia. In R. G. Heimberg & M. R. Liebowitz (Eds.), *Social phobia: Diagnosis, assessment, and treatment* (pp. 94–112). New York: Guilford Press.

Lenzinger, E., Neumeister, A., Praschak-Rieder, N., Fuchs, K., Gerhard, E., Willeit, M., et al. (1999). Behavioral effects of tryptophan depletion in seasonal affective disorder associated with the serotonin transporter gene? *Psychiatry Research, 85*, 241–246.

Leonhard, K. (1979). *The classification of endogenous psychoses.* New York : Irvington.

Lesch, K. P., Bengel, D., Heils, A., Sabol, S. Z., Greenberg, B. D., Petri, S., Benjamin, J., Muller, C. R., Hamer, D. H., & Murphy, D. L. (1996). Selective alteration of personality and social behavior by serotonergic intervention. *Science, 274*, 1527–1531.

Lewis, C. E., & Bucholz, K. (1991). Alcoholism, antisocial behavior and family history. *British Journal of Addiction, 86*, 177–194.

Lewis, D. A., & Levitt, P. (2002). Schizophrenia as a disorder of neurodevelopment. *Annual Review of Neuroscience, 25*, 409–432.

Linney, Y. M., Murray, R. M., Peters, E. R., MacDonald, A. M., Rijsdijk, F., & Sham, P. C. (2003). A quantitative genetic analysis of schizotypal personality traits. *Psychological Medicine, 33*, 803–816.

Livesley, W. J. (1985a). The classification of personality disorder: I. The choice of category concept. *Canadian Journal of Psychiatry, 30*, 353–358.

Livesley, W. J. (1985b). The classification of personality disorder: II. The problem of criteria. *Canadian Journal of Psychiatry, 30*, 359–362.

Livesley, W. J. (1986). Trait and behavioral prototypes of personality disorder. *American Journal of Psychiatry, 143*, 728–732.

Livesley, W. J. (1999). The implications of recent research on the etiology and stability of personality and personality disorder for treatment. In J. Derksen, C. Maffei, & H. Groen (Eds.), *The treatment of personality disorders* (pp. 35–37). New York: Plenum Press.

Livesley, W. J. (2001). Framework for an integrated approach to treatment. In W. J. Livesley (Ed.), *Handbook of personality disorder* (pp. 570–600). New York: Guilford Press.

Livesley, W. J., Jackson, D. N., & Schroeder, M. L. (1989). A study of the factorial structure of personality pathology. *Journal of Personality Disorders, 3*, 292–306.

Livesley, W. J., & Jackson, D. N. (in press). *Manual for the Dimensional Assessment of Personality Pathology-Basic Questionnaire (DAPP).* London, Ontario: Research Psychologists' Press.

Livesley, W. J., Jang, K. L., & Vernon, P. A. (1998). Phenotypic and genetic structure of traits delineating personality disorder. *Archives of General Psychiatry, 55*, 941–948.

Loehlin, J. C., & Nichols, R. C. (1976). *Heredity, environment, and personality: A study of 850 sets of twins.* Austin: University of Texas Press.

Loehlin, J. C. (1982). Are personality traits differentially heritable? *Behavior Genetics, 12*, 417–428.

Loehlin, J. C. (1986). Are California Psychological Inventory items differentially heritable? *Behavior Genetics, 16*, 599–603.

Loehlin, J. C. (1992). *Genes and environment in personality development.* Newbury Park, CA: Sage.

Loehlin, J. C., Horn, J. M., & Willermann, L. (1997). Heredity, environment, and IQ in the Texas adoption study. In R. J. Sternberg, & E. L. Grigorenko (Eds.), *Heredity, Environment, and Intelligence* (pp. 105–125). New York: Cambridge University Press.

Loftus, E. F., & Pickrell, J. E.(1995). The formation of false memories. *Psychiatric Annals, 25*, 720–725.

Loftus, J., Delisi, L. E., & Crow, T. J. (2000). Factor structure and familiality of first-rank symptoms in sibling pairs with schizophrenia and schizoaffective disorder. *British Journal of Psychiatry, 177*, 15–19.

Lusher, J., Ebersole, L., & Ball, D. (2000). Dopamine D4 receptor gene and severity of dependence. *Addiction Biology, 5*, 471–474.

Lyons, M. J., Eisen, S. A., Goldberg, J., True, W., Lin, N., Meyer, J. M., et al. (1998). A registry-based twin study of depression in men. *Archives of General Psychiatry, 5*, 468–472.

Lyons, M. J., True, W. R., Eisen, S. A., & Goldberg, J. (1995). Differential heritability of adult and juvenile antisocial traits. *Archives of General Psychiatry, 52*, 906–915.

Macaskill, G. T., Hopper, J. L., White, V., & Hill, D. J. (1994). Genetic and environmental variation in Eysenck Personality scales measured on Australian adolescent twins. *Behavior Genetics, 24*, 481–491.

Madden, P. A., Heath, A. C., Rosenthal, N. E., & Martin, N. G. (1996). Seasonal changes in mood and behavior. The role of genetic factors. *Archives of General Psychiatry, 53*, 47–55.

Maes, M., Meltzer, H. Y., Scharpe, S., & Bosmans, E. (1993). Relationships between lower plasma L-tryptophan levels and immune-inflammatory variables in depression. *Psychiatry Research, 49*, 151–165.

Maier, W., & Buller, R. (1988) One-year follow-up of panic disorder: Outcome and prognostic factors. *European Archive of Psychiatry and Clinical Neuroscience, 238*, 105–109.

Malhotra, A. K., Goldman, D., Ozaki, N., & Breier, A. (1996). Lack of association between polymorphisms in the 5-HT-sub(2A) receptor gene and the antipsychotic response to clozapine. *American Journal of Psychiatry, 153*, 1092–1094.

Mannuzza, S., Schneier, F. R., Chapman, T. F., Liebowitz, M. R., Klein, D. F., & Fyer, A. J. (1995). Generalized social phobia: Reliability and validity. *Archives of General Psychiatry, 5*, 230–237.

Marenco, S., & Weinberger, D. R. (2000). The neurodevelopmental hypothesis of schizophrenia: Following a trail of evidence from cradle to grave. *Development and Psychopathology. 12*, 501–527.

Markon, K. E., Krueger, R. F., Bouchard, T. J., Jr., & Gottesman, I. I. (2002). Normal and abnormal personality traits: Evidence for genetic and environmental relationships in the Minnesota Study of Twins Reared Apart. *Journal of Personality, 70*, 661–694.

Martin, N. G., Boomsma, D. I., & Machin, M. A. (1997, December). A twin pronged attack on complex traits. *Nature Genetics, 17*, 387–392.

Martin, S. D., Martin, E., Rai, S. S., Richardson, M. A., & Royall, R. (2001). Brain blood flow changes in depressed patients treated with interpersonal psychotherapy or venlafaxine hydrochloride: Preliminary findings. *Archives of General Psychiatry, 58*, 641–648.

Mason, O., Claridge, G., & Jackson, M. (1995). New scales for the assessment of schizotypy. *Personality and Individual Differences, 18*, 7–13.

Mauricio, M., O'Hara, R., Yesavage, J. A., Friedman, L., Kraemer, H. C., Van De Water, M., et al. (2000). A longitudinal study of Apolipoprotein-E genotype and depressive symptoms in community-dwelling older adults. *American Journal of Geriatric Psychiatry, 8*, 196–200.

Mavissakalian, M. (1985). Male and female agoraphobia: Are they different? *Behavior Research and Therapy, 23,* 469–471.

Mayberg, H. S., Brannan, S. K., Mahurin, R. K., Jerabek, P. A., Brickman, J. S., et al. (1997). Cingulate function in depression: A potential predictor of treatment response. *NeuroReport, 8,* 1057–1061.

McClearn, G. E., Plomin, R., Gora-Maslak, G., & Crabbe, J. C. (1991). The gene chase in behavioral science. *Psychological Science, 2,* 222–229.

McCrae, R. R., Jang, K. L, Livesley, W. J., Riemann, R., & Angleitner, A. (2001). Sources of structure: Genetic, environmental, and artifactual influences on the covariance of personality traits. *Journal of Personality, 69,* 511–535.

McDougle, C. J., Epperson, C. N., Price, L. H., & Gelernter, J. (1998). Evidence for linkage disequilibrium between serotonin transporter protein gene (SLC6A4) and obsessive compulsive disorder. *Molecular Psychiatry, 3,* 270–273.

McGue, M., Pickens, R. W., Svikis, D. S. (1992). Sex and age effects on the inheritance of alcohol problems: A twin study. *Journal of Abnormal Psychology, 101,* 3–17.

McGue, M., Slutske, W., Taylor, J., & Iancono, W. G. (1997). Personality and substance use disorders: I. Effects of gender and alcoholism subtype. *Alcoholism: Clinical and Experimental Research, 21,* 513–520.

McGuffin, P., Katz, R., Watkins, S., & Rutherford, J. (1996). A hospital-based twin register of the heritability of *DSM-IV* unipolar depression. *Archives of General Psychiatry, 53,* 129–136.

McGuffin, P., & Thapar, A. (1992). The genetics of personality disorder. *British Journal of Psychiatry, 160,* 12–23.

McNeil, T. F., Cantor-Graae, E., & Weinberger, D. R. (2000). Relationship of obstetric complications and differences in size of brain structures in monozygotic twin pairs discordant for schizophrenia. *American Journal of Psychiatry, 157,* 203–212.

Meehl, P. E. (1962). Schizotaxia, schizotypy schizophrenia. *American Psychologist, 17,* 827–831.

Meehl, P. E. (1989) Schizotaxia revisited. *Archives of General Psychiatry, 46,* 935–944.

Merikangas, K. R., & Avenevoli, S. (2000). Implications of genetic epidemiology for the prevention of substance use disorders. *Addictive Behaviors, 25,* 807–820.

Millon, T. (1996). Avoidant personality disorder. In: T. A. Widiger, A. J. Frances, H. A. Pincus, R. Ross, M. B. First, & W. W. Davis (Eds.), *DSM sourcebook* (Vol. 2, pp. 757–766). Washington, DC: American Psychiatric Publishing.

Mineka, S., Watson, D., & Clark, L. A. (1998). Comorbidity of anxiety and mood disorders. *Annual Review of Psychology, 49,* 377–412.

Moises, H. W., Yang, L., Kristbjarnarson, H., Wiese, C., Byerley, W., Macciardi, F., et al. (1995). An international two-stage genome-wide search for schizophrenia susceptibility genes. *Nature Genetics, 11,* 321–324.

Moises, H. W., Yang, L., Li, T., Havsteen, B., Fimmers, R., Baur, M. P., et al. (1995). Potential linkage disequilibrium between schizophrenia and locus D22S278 on the long arm of chromosome 22. *American Journal of Medical Genetics, 60,* 465–467.

Moos, R. H., & Moos, B. S. (1974). *Classroom Environment Scale (CES).* Palo Alto, CA: Consulting Psychologists Press.

Moos, R. H., & Moos, B. S. (1986). *Family Environment Scale.* Palo Alto, NM: Consulting Psychologists Press.

Moos, R. H., & Moos, B. S. (1994). *Family Environment Scale* (2nd ed.). Alto, NM: Consulting Psychologists Press.

Murphy, G. M., Jr., Kremer, C., Rodrigues, H. E., & Schatzberg, A. F. (2003). Pharmacogenetics of antidepressant medication intolerance. *Journal of Psychiatry, 160,* 1830–1835.

Muscettola, G., Barbato, G., Ficca, G., Beatrice, M., Puca, M., Aguglia, E., et al. (1995). Seasonality of mood in Italy: Role of latitude and sociocultural factors. *Journal of Affective Disorders, 33,* 135–139.

Nathan, P. E., & Gorman, J. M. (Eds) (2002). *A guide to treatments that work* (2nd ed.). Oxford, England: Oxford University Press.

Neale, M. C. & Cardon, L. R. (1992). *Methodology for genetic studies of twins and families.* Dordrecht: Kluwer.

Nelson, E. C., Cloninger, C. R., Przybeck, T. R, & Csernansky, J. G. (1996). Platelet serotonergic markers and tridimensional personality questionnaire measures in a clinical sample. *Biological Psychiatry, 40,* 271–278.

Nestadt, G., Samuels, J., Riddle, M. A., Liang, K. Y., Bienvenu, O. J., Hoehn-Saric, R., et al. (2001). The relationship between obsessive-compulsive disorder and anxiety and affective disorders: Results from the Johns Hopkins OCD Family Study. *Psychological Medicine, 31,* 481–487.

Nestadt, G., Lan, T., Samuels, J., Riddle, M., Bienvenu, O. J., III, Liang, K. Y., et al. (2000). Complex segregation analysis provides compelling evidence for a major gene underlying obsessive-compulsive disorder and for heterogeneity by sex. *American Journal of Human Genetics, 6,* 1611–1616.

Nigg, J. T., & Goldsmith, H. H. (1994). Genetics of personality disorders: Perspectives from personality and psychopathology research. *Psychological Bulletin, 115,* 346–380.

Noyes, R., Jr., Clarkson, C., Crowe, R. R., Yates, W. R., & McChesney, C. M. (1987). A family study of generalized anxiety disorder. *American Journal of Psychiatry, 144,* 1019–1024.

Oei, T. P., Wanstall, K., & Evans, L. (1990). Sex differences in panic disorder with agoraphobia. *Journal of Anxiety Disorders, 4,* 317–324.

Ohtsuki, T., Toru, M., & Arinami, T. (2001). Mutation screening of the metabotropic glutamate receptor mGluR4 (GRM4) gene in patients with schizophrenia. *Psychiatric Genetics, 11,* 79–83.

Okawa, M., Shirakawa, S., Uchiyama, M., Oguri, M., Kohsaka, M., & Mishima, K. (1996). Seasonal variation of mood and behavior in a healthy middle aged population in Japan. *Acta Psychiatrica Scandinavica, 94,* 211–216.

Olson, J. M., Vernon, P. A., Harris, J. A., & Jang, K. L. (2001). The heritability of attitudes: A study of twins. *Journal of Personality and Social Psychology, 806,* 845–860.

Ono, Y., Yoshimura, K., Mizushima, H., Manki, H., Yagi, G., Kanba, S., et al. (1999). Environmental and possible genetic contributions to character dimensions of personality. *Psychological Reports, 84,* 689–696.

Paris, J. (1994). *Borderline personality disorder: A multidimensional approach.* Washington, DC: American Psychiatric Association.

Paris, J. (1996). *Social factors in the personality disorders.* New York: Cambridge University Press.

Paris, J. (2001). Psychosocial adversity. In W. J. Livesley (Ed.), *Handbook of personality disorders: Theory, research, and treatment* (pp. 231–241). New York: Guilford Press.

Parker, G., Tupling, H., & Brown, L. B. (1979). A parental bonding instrument. *British Journal of Medical Psychology, 52,* 1–10.

Passini, F. T., & Norman, W. T. (1966). A universal conception of personality structure? *Journal of Personality and Social Psychology, 4,* 44–49.

Pauls, D. L., Alsobrook, J. P., II, Goodman, W., Rasmussen, S., & Leckman, J. F. (1995). A family study of obsessive compulsive disorder. *American Journal of Psychiatry, 152,* 76–84.

Pedersen, W., & Skrondal, A. (1998). Alcohol consumption debut: Predictors and consequences. *Journal of Studies on Alcohol, 59,* 32–42.

Perna, G., Cocchi, S., & Bertani, A. (1995). Sensitivity to 35% CO-sub-2 in healthy first-degree relatives of patients with panic disorder. *American Journal of Psychiatry, 152,* 623–625.

Perna, G., Bertani, A., Caldirola, D., & Bellodi, L. (1996). Family history of panic disorder and hypersensitivity to CO2 in patients with panic disorder. *American Journal of Psychiatry, 153,* 1060–1064.

Peters, E. R., Joseph, S. A., & Garety, P. A. (1999). Measurement of delusional ideation in the normal population: Introducing the PDI. *Schizophrenia Bulletin, 25,* 553–576.

Peterson, R. A., & Reiss, S. (1992). *Anxiety Sensitivity Index manual* (2nd ed., rev.). Worthington, OH: International Diagnostic Systems.

Plomin, R., DeFries, J. C., & Loehlin, J. C. (1977). Genotype-environment interaction and correlation in the analysis of human behavior. *Psychological Bulletin, 84,* 309–322.

Plomin, R., DeFries, J. C., & McClearn, G. E. (1990). *Behavioral genetics: A primer* (2nd ed.). New York: Freeman.

Plomin, R., Rende, R., & Rutter, M. (1991).Quantitative genetics and developmental psychopathology. In D. Cicchetti, & S. L. Toth (Eds.), *Internalizing and externalizing expressions of dysfunction: RochesterSymposium on Developmental Psychopathology* (Vol. 2, pp. 155–202). Hillsdale, NJ: Lawrence Erlbaum Associates.

Plomin, R., & Caspi, A. (1998). DNA and personality. *European Journal of Personality, 12,* 387–407.

Plomin, R., DeFries, J. C., & McClearn, G. E. (2000). *Behavioral genetics: A primer* (4th ed.). New York: Freeman.

Plomin, R., & Crabbe, J. (2000). DNA. *Psychological Bulletin, 126,* 806–828.

Plomin, R., DeFries, J. C., Craig, I. W., & McGuffin, P. (Eds.). (2003). *Behavioral genetics in the postgenomic era.* Washington, DC: American Psychological Association.

Pogue-Geile, M., Ferrell, R., Deka, R., Debski, T., & Manuck, S. (1998). Human novelty-seeking personality traits and dopamine D4 receptor polymorphisms: A twin and genetic association study. *American Journal of Medical Genetics, 81,* 44–48.

Prabhu, V. R., Porjesz, B., Chorlian, D. B., Wang, K., Stimus, A., & Begleiter, H. (2001). Visual P3 in female alcoholics. *Alcoholism: Clinical and Experimental Research, 25,* 531–539.

Prescott, C. A., Aggen, S. H., & Kendler, K. S. (2000). Sex-specific genetic influences on the comorbidity of alcoholism and major depression in a population-based sample of US twins. *Archives of General Psychiatry, 57,* 803–811.

Prescott, C. A., Hewitt, J. K., Truett, K. R., & Heath, A. C. (1994). Genetic and environmental influences on lifetime alcohol-related problems in a volunteer sample of older twins. *Journal of Studies on Alcohol, 55,* 184–202.

Prescott, C. A., & Kendler, K. S. (1999). Genetic and environmental contributions to alcohol abuse and dependence in a population-based sample of male twins. *American Journal of Psychiatry, 156,* 34–40.

Prescott, C. A., & Kendler, K. S.(1996). Longitudinal stability and change in alcohol consumption among female twins: Contributions of genetics. *Development and Psychopathology, 8,* 849–866.

Purcell, S. (2002). Variance components models for gene-environment interaction in twin analysis. *Twin Research, 5,* 554–571.

Pulver, A. E., Lasseter, V. K., Kasch, L., Wolyniec, P., Nestadt, G., Blouin, J. L., et al. (1995). Schizophrenia: A genome scan targets chromosomes 3p and 8p as potential sites of susceptibility genes. *American Journal of Medical Genetics, 60,* 252–260.

Radant, A., Tsuang, D., Peskind, E. R., McFall, M., & Raskind, W. (2001). Biological markers and diagnostic accuracy in the genetics of posttraumatic stress disorder. *Psychiatry Research, 102,* 203–215.

Radloff, L. S . (1977). The CES-D scale: A new self-report depression scale for research in the general population. *Applied Psychological Measurement, 1,* 385–401.

Rapee, R. M., & Heimberg, R. G. (1997). A cognitive-behavioral model of anxiety in social phobia. *Behavior Research and Therapy, 35,* 741–756.

Reddy, P. S., Reddy, Y. C., Srinath, S., Khanna, S., Sheshadri, S. P., & Girimaji, S. R. (2001). A family study of juvenile obsessive-compulsive disorder. *Canadian Journal of Psychiatry-Revue Canadienne de Psychiatrie, 46,* 346–351.

Ridley, M. (2003). *Nature via nurture: Genes, experience, and what makes us human.* New York: Harper Collins.

Riemann, R., Angleitner, A., & Strelau, J. (1997). Genetic and environmental influences on personality: A study of twins reared together using the self- and peer-report NEO-FFI scales. *Journal of Personality, 65,* 449–475.

Riggins-Caspers, K., Cadoret, R. J., Panak, W., Lempers, J. D., Troughton, E., & Stewart, M. A. (1999). Gene-environment interaction and the moderating effect of adoption agency disclosure on estimating genetic effects. *Personality and Individual Differences, 27,* 357–380.

Rose, R. J. (1988). Genetic and environmental variance in content dimensions of the MMPI. *Journal of Personality and Social Psychology, 55,* 302–311.

Rose, R. J., Kaprio, J., Winter, T., Koskenvuo, M., & Viken, R. J. (1999). Familial and socioregional environmental effects on abstinence from alcohol at age sixteen. *Journal of Studies on Alcohol* (Supp. 13), 63–74.

Rose, R. J., Dick, D. M., Viken, R. J., Pulkkinen, L., &Kaprio, J. (2001). Drinking or abstaining at age 14? A genetic epidemiological study. *Alcoholism: Clinical and Experimental Research, 25,* 1594–1604.

Rosen, L. N., Targum, S. D., Terman, M., Bryant, M. J., Hoffman, H., Kasper, S. F., et al. (1990). Prevalence of seasonal affective disorder at four latitudes. *Psychiatry Research, 31,* 131–144.

Rosenthal, N. E., Mazzanti, C. M., Barnett, R. L., Hardin, T. A., Turner, E. H., Lam, G. K., et al. (1998). Role of serotonin transporter promoter repeat length polymorphism (5-HTTLPR) in seasonality and seasonal affective disorder. *Molecular Psychiatry, 3,* 175–177.

Rosenthal, N. E., & Wehr, T. A. (1987). Seasonal affective disorders. *Psychiatric Annals, 17,* 670–674.

Roy, M. A., Neale, M. C., Pedersen, N. L., Mathé, A. A., & Kendler, K. S. (1995). A twin study of generalized anxiety disorder and major depression. *Psychological Medicine, 25,* 1037–1049.

Rutter, M. (1987). Temperament, personality, and personality disorder. *British Journal of Psychiatry, 150,* 443–458.

Rutter, M. (1989). Pathways from childhood to adult life. *Journal of Child Psychology and Psychiatry and Allied Disciplines, 30,* 23–51.

Rutter, M. (2002). Nature, nurture, and development: From evangelism through science toward policy and practice. *Child Development, 73,* 1–21.

Rutter, M. (2003). Genetic Influences on risk and protection: Implications for understanding resilience. In S. S. Luthar (Ed.), 2003. *Resilience and vulnerability: Adaptation in the context of childhood adversities* (pp. 489–509). New York: Cambridge University Press.

Saucier, G., & Goldberg, L. R. (1996). The language of personality: Lexical perspectives on the five-factor model. In J. S. Wiggins (Ed.), *The five factor model of personality* (pp. 21–50). New York: Guilford Press.

Saudino, K. J., Pedersen, N. L., Lichtenstein, P., & McClearn, G. E. (1997). Can personality explain genetic influences on life events? *Journal of Personality and Social Psychology, 72,* 196–206.

Schneider, K. (1959). *Clinical psychopathology* (5th ed., M. W. Hamilton, Trans.). Oxford, England: Grune and Stratton. (Original work published 1959)

Schuckit, M. A., Klein, J., Twitchell, G., & Smith, T. L. (1994). Personality test scores as predictors of alcoholism almost a decade later. *American Journal of Psychiatry, 151,* 1038–1042.

Schuckit, M. A. (1983). Alcoholism and other psychiatric disorders. *Hospital and Community Psychiatry, 34,* 1022–1027.

Schwab, S. G., Hallmayer, J., Lerer, B., Albus, M., Borrmann, M., & Honing, S. (1998). Support for a chromosome 18p locus conferring susceptibility to functional psychoses in families with schizophrenia, by association and linkage analysis. *American Journal of Human Genetics, 63,* 1139–1152.

Seligman, M. E. (1971). Phobias and preparedness. *Behavior Therapy, 2,* 307–320.

Seroczynski, A. D., Bergeman, C. S., & Coccaro, E. F. (1999). Etiology of the impulsivity/aggression relationship: Genes or environment? *Psychiatry Research, 86,* 41–57.

Serretti, A., Benedetti, F., Colombo, C., Lilli, R., Lorenzi, C., & Smeraldi, E. (1999). Dopamine receptor D4 is not associated with antidepressant activity of sleep deprivation. *Psychiatry Research, 89,* 107–114.

Seidman, S. N., Araujo, A. B., Roose, S. P., & McKinlay, J. B. (2001). Testosterone level, androgen receptor polymorphism, and depressive symptoms in middle-aged men. *Biological Psychiatry, 50,* 371–376.

Sham, P. C., Sterne, A., Purcell, S., Cherney, S., Webster, M., & Rijsdik, F.(2000). GENESiS: Creating a composite index of the vulnerability to anxiety and depression in a community-based sample of siblings. *Twin Research, 3,* 316–322.

Sher, K. J., & Trull, T. J. (1994). Personality and disinhibitory psychopathology: Alcoholism and antisocial personality disorder. *Journal of Abnormal Psychology, 103,* 92–102.

Silverman, J. M., Smith, C. J., Guo, S. L., Mohs, R. C., Siever, L. J., & Davis, K. L. (1998). Lateral ventricular enlargement in schizophrenic probands and their siblings with schizophrenia-related disorders. *Biological Psychiatry, 43,* 97–106.

Slutske, W. S., Heath, A. C., Madden, P. A. F., Bucholz, K. K., Statham, D. J., & Martin, N. G. (2002). Personality and the genetic risk for alcohol dependence. *Journal of Abnormal Psychology, 111,* 124–133.

Smoller, J. W., Pollack, M. H., Otto, M. W., Rosenbaum, J. F., & Kradin, R. L. (1996). Panic anxiety, dyspnea, and respiratory disease: Theoretical and clinical considerations. *American Journal of Respiratory and Critical Care Medicine, 154,* 6–17.

Spitzer, R. L., Endicott, J., & Robins, E. (1978). Research diagnostic criteria: Rationale and reliability. *Archives of General Psychiatry, 35,* 773–782.

Spitzer, R., Endicott, J., & Gibbon, M. (1979). Crossing the border into borderline personality disorder and borderline schizophrenia: The development of criteria. *Archives of General Psychiatry, 36,* 17–24.

Stancer, H. C., Persad, E., Wagener, D. K., & Jorna, T. (1987). Evidence for homogeneity of major depression and bipolar affective disorder. *Journal of Psychiatric Research, 21,* 37–53.

Steffens, D. C., Plassman, B. L., Helms, M. J., Welsh-Bohmer, K. A., Saunders, A. M., & Breitner, J. C. (1997). A twin study of late-onset depression and apolipoprotein E epsilon 4 as risk factors for Alzheimer's disease. *Biological Psychiatry, 41,* 851–856.

Stein, M. B., Walker, J. R., Anderson, G., Hazen, A. L., Ross, C. A., Eldridge, G., et al. (1996). Childhood physical and sexual abuse in patients with anxiety disorders and in a community sample. *American Journal of Psychiatry, 153,* 275–277.

Stein, M. B., Jang, K. L., & Livesley, W. J. (1999). Heritability of anxiety sensitivity: A twin study. *American Journal of Psychiatry, 156,* 246–251.

Stein, M. B., Chartier, M. J., Kozak, M. V., King, N., & Kennedy, J. L. (1998). Genetic linkage to the serotonin transporter protein and 5HT2A receptor genes excluded in generalized social phobia. *Psychiatry Research, 81,* 283–291.

Stein, M. B., Jang, K. L., Taylor, S., Vernon, P. A. & Livesley, W. J. (2002). Genetic and environmental influences on trauma exposure and posttraumatic stress disorder symptoms: A twin study. *American Journal of Psychiatry, 159,* 1675–1681.

Stein, M. B., Chartier, M. J., Hazen, A. L., Kozak, M. V., Tancer, M. E., Lader, S., et al. (1998). A direct-interview family study of generalized social phobia. *American Journal of Psychiatry, 155,* 90–97.

Stein, M. B., Jang, K. L. & Livesley, W. J. (2002). Heritability of social anxiety-related concerns and personality characteristics: A twin study. *Journal of Nervous and Mental Disease, 190,* 219–224.

Stein, M. B., Chartier, M. J., Kozak, M. V., & Jang, K. L. (2001). Familial aggregation of anxiety-related quantitative traits in generalized social phobia: Clues to understanding "disorder" heritability? *American Journal of Medical Genetics, 105,* 79–83.

Stein, M. B., & Chavira, D. A. (1998). Subtypes of social phobia and comorbidity with depression and other anxiety disorders. *Journal of Affective Disorders, 50,* (S1) S11–S16.

Stewart, R., Russ, C., & Richards, M. (2001). Depression, APOE genotype and subjective memory impairment: A cross-sectional study in an African-Caribbean population. *Psychological Medicine, 31,* 431–440.

Stewart, S. H., Taylor, S., & Baker, J. M. (1990). Gender differences in dimensions of anxiety sensitivity. *Journal of Anxiety Disorders, 11,* 179–200.

Stopa, L., & Clark, D. M. (2000). Social phobia and interpretation of social events. *Behavior Research and Therapy, 38,* 273–283.

Straub, R. E., MacLean, C. J., O'Neill, F. A., Burke, J., Murphy, B., & Duke, F. (1995). A potential vulnerability locus for schizophrenic on chromosome 6p22-24: Evidence for genetic heterogeneity. *Nature Genetics, 11,* 287–293.

Sullivan, P. F., Neale, M. C., & Kendler, K. S. (2000). Genetic epidemiology of major depression: Review and meta-analysis. *American Journal of Psychiatry, 157,* 1552–1562.

Sullivan, P. F., Kendler, K. S., & Neale, M. C. (2003). Schizophrenia as a complex trait: evidence from a meta-analysis of twin studies. *Archives of General Psychiatry, 60,* 1187–1192.

Sulloway, F. J. (1995). Birth order and evolutionary psychology: A meta-analytic overview. *Psychological Inquiry, 6,* 75–80.

Syagailo, Y. V., Stober, G., Grassle, M., Reimer, E., Knapp, M., Jungkunz, G., et al. (2001). Association analysis of the functional monoamine oxidase A gene promoter polymorphism in psychiatric disorders. *American Journal of Medical Genetics, 105,* 168–171.

Taylor, S. (1995). Anxiety sensitivity: Theoretical perspectives and recent findings. *Behavior Research and Therapy, 33,* 243–258.

Tellegen, A. (1982). *Brief manual for the Differential Personality Questionnaire.* Unpublished manuscript, University of Minnesota, Minneapolis.

Temple, L. K., McLeod, R. S., Gallinger, S., & Wright, J. G. (2001, August 3). Essays on science and society: Defining disease in the genomics era. *Science, 293,* 807–808.

Tennant, C. (1988). Parental loss in childhood: Its effect in adult life. *Archives of General Psychiatry, 45,* 1045–1050.

Thapar, A., & McGuffin, P. (1993). Is personality disorder inherited? An overview of the evidence. *Journal of Psychopathology and Behavioral Assessment, 15,* 325–345.

Tiihonen J., Hallikainen T., Lachman H., Saito T., Volavka J., Kauhanen J., et al. (1999). Association between the functional variant of the catechol-O-methyltransferase (COMT) gene and type 1 alcoholism. *Molecular Psychiatry, 4,* 286–289.

Tooby, J., & Cosmides, L. (1990). On the universality of human nature and the uniqueness of the individual: The role of genetics and adaptation. *Journal of Personality, 58,* 17–67.

Torgersen, S., Skre, I., Onstad, S., Edvardsen, J., & Kringlen, E. (1993). The psychometric-genetic structure of DSM-III-R personality disorder criteria. *Journal of Personality Disorders, 7,* 196–213.

Torgersen, S., Lygren, S., & Oien, P. A. (2000). A twin study of personality disorders. *Comprehensive Psychiatry, 41*, 416–425.

Trivers, R. (1985). *Social evolution*. Menlo Park, CA: Benjamin Cummings.

True, W. R., Rice, J., Eisen, S. A., Heath, A. C., Goldberg, J., Lyons, M. J., et al. (1993). A twin study of genetic and environmental contributions to liability for posttraumatic stress symptoms. *Archives of General Psychiatry, 50*, 257–264.

Tsuang, M. T. (2001). Defining alternative phenotypes for genetic studies: What can we learn from studies of schizophrenia?. *American Journal of Medical Genetics, 105*, 8–10.

Tsuang, M. T., Lyons, M. J., Meyer, J. M., Doyle, T., Eisen, S. A., Goldberg, J., et al. (1998). Co-occurrence of abuse of different drugs in men: The role of drug-specific and shared vulnerabilities. *Archives of General Psychiatry, 55*, 967–972.

Tsuang, M. T., Stone, W. S., & Faraone, S. V. (1999). The genetics of schizophrenia. *Current Psychiatry Reports, 1*, 20–24.

Tsuang, M. T., Stone, W. S., Seidman, L. J., Faraone, S. V., Zimmet, S., Wojcik, J., et al. (1999). Treatment of nonpsychotic relatives of patients with schizophrenia: Four case studies. *Biological Psychiatry, 45*, 1412–1418.

Tsuang, M. T., Stone, W. S., & Faraone, S. V. (2002). Understanding predisposition to schizophrenia: Toward intervention and prevention. *Canadian Journal of Psychiatry-Revue Canadienne de Psychiatrie, 47*, 518–526.

Turkheimer, E., & Waldron, M. (2000). Nonshared environment: A theoretical, methodological, and quantitative review. *Psychological Bulletin, 126*, 78–108.

Tyrer, P. (1999). Borderline personality disorder: A motley diagnosis in need of reform. *Lancet, 354*, 1095–1096.

Uhl, G. R., & Grow, R. W. (2004). The burden of complex genetics in brain disorders. *Archives of General Psychiatry, 61*, 223–229.

Vanakoski, J., Virkkunen, M., Naukkarinen, H., & Goldman, D. (2001). No association of CCK and CCK-sub(B) receptor polymorphisms with alcohol dependence. *Psychiatry Research, 102*, 1–7.

Vandenbergh, D. J., Zonderman, A. B., Wang, J., Uhl, G. R., & Costa, P. T. (1997). No association between Novelty Seeking and dopamine D4 receptor (DRD4) exon III seven repeat alleles in Baltimore Longitudinal Study of Aging participants. *Molecular Psychiatry, 2*, 417–419.

Van Kampen, D. (1999). Genetic and environmental influences on pre-schizophrenic personality: MAXCOV-HITMAX and LISREL analyses. *European Journal of Personality, 13*, 63–80.

van Velzen, C. J., Emmelkamp, P. M., & Scholing, A. (2000). Generalized social phobia versus avoidant personality disorder: Differences in psychopathology, personality traits, and social and occupational functioning. *Journal of Anxiety Disorders, 14*, 395–411.

Vernon, P. A., McCarthy, J. M., Johnson, A. M., Jang, K. L., & Harris, J. A. (1999). Individual differences in multiple dimensions of aggression: a univariate and multivariate genetic analysis. *Twin Research, 2*, 16–21.

Vollebergh, W. A. M ., Ledema, J., Bijl, R. V., de Graaf, R., Smitt, F., & Ormel, J. (2001). The structure and stability of common mental disorders: The NEMESIS Study. *Archives of General Psychiatry, 58*, 597–603.

Wade, T. D., Bulik, C. M., Neale, M., & Kendler, K. S. (2000). Anorexia nervosa and major depression: Shared genetic and environmental risk factors. *American Journal of Psychiatry, 157*, 469–471.

Wahlberg, K. E., Wynne, L. C., Oja, H., Keskitalo, P., Pykalainen, L., Lahti, I., et al. (1997). Gene-environment interaction in vulnerability to schizophrenia: Findings from the Finnish Adoptive Family Study of Schizophrenia. *American Journal of Psychiatry, 154*, 355–362.

Waller, N. G., & Shaver, P. R. (1994). The importance of nongenetic influences on romantic love styles: A twin-family study. *Psychological Science, 5*, 268–274.

Watson, D., & Friend, R. (1969). Measurement of social-evaluative anxiety. *Journal of Consulting and Clinical Psychology, 33,* 448–457.

Watt, M. C., Stewart, S. H., & Cox, B. J. (1998). A retrospective study of the learning history origins of anxiety sensitivity. *Behavior Research and Therapy, 36,* 505–525.

Weinberg, R. A. (1989). Intelligence and IQ: Landmark issues and great debates. *American Psychologist, 44,* 98–104.

Weinberger, D. R. (1987). Implications of normal brain development for the pathogenesis of schizophrenia. *Archives of General Psychiatry, 44,* 660–669.

Weissman, M. M., Fyer, A. J., Haghighi, F., Heiman, G., Deng, Z., Hen, R.,et al. (2000). Potential panic disorder syndrome: Clinical and genetic linkage evidence. *American Journal of Medical Genetics, 96,* 24–35.

Werner, E. E., & Smith, R. S. (1992). *Overcoming the odds: High risk children from birth to adulthood.* Ithaca, NY: Cornell University Press.

White, C. N., Gunderson, J. G., & Zanarini, M. C. (2003). Family studies of borderline personality disorder: A review. *Harvard Review of Psychiatry, 11,* 8–19.

White, D. M., Lewy, A. J., Sack, R. J., & Blood, M. L. (1990). Is winter depression a bipolar disorder? *Comprehensive Psychiatry, 31,* 196–204.

Widiger, T. A. (1998). Four out of five ain't bad. *Archives of General Psychiatry, 55,* 865–866.

Widiger, T. A. (2003). Personality disorder and Axis I psychopathology: The problematic boundary of Axis I and Axis II. *Journal of Personality Disorders, 17,* 90–108.

Widiger, T. A., Verheul, R., & van den Brink, W. (1999). Personality and psychopathology. In L. A. Pervin, & O. P. John (Eds.), *Handbook of personality: Theory and research* (2nd ed., pp. 347–366). New York: Guilford Press.

Wiggins, J. S. (1966). Substantive dimensions of self-report in the MMPI item pool. *Psychological Monographs: General and Applied, 80,* 42.

Willeit, M., Praschak-Rieder, N., Neumeister, A., Pirker, W., Asenbaum, S., Vitouch, O., et al. (2000). 23I-beta-CIT SPECT imaging shows reduced brain serotonin transporter availability in drug-free depressed patients with seasonal affective disorder. *Biological Psychiatry, 47,* 482–489.

Wilson, S. E., Bell, R. W., & Arredondo, R. (1995). Temperament, family environment, and family history of alcohol abuse. *Alcoholism Treatment Quarterly, 12,* 55–68.

Wirz-Justice, A., Bucheli, C., Schmid, A. C., & Graw, P. (1986). A dose relationship in bright white light treatment of seasonal depression. *American Journal of Psychiatry, 143,* 932–933.

World Health Organization. (1967). *International classification of diseases injuries and causes of death: 8th revision.* Geneva, Switzerland: World Health Organization (WHO).

World Health Organization (1992). *The ICD-10 classification of mental and behavioral disorders: Clinical descriptions and diagnostic guidelines.* Geneva, Switzerland: World Health Organization (WHO).

Wright, P., Nimgaonkar, V. L., Donaldson, P. T., & Murray, R. M. (2001). Schizophrenia and HLA: A review. *Schizophrenia Research, 47,* 1–12.

Wright, S. (1960). Path coefficients and path regressions: Alternative or complementary concepts? *Biometrics, 16,* 189–202.

Young, S. E., Stallings, M. C., Corley, R. P., Krauter, K. S., & Hewitt, J. K. (2000). Genetic and environmental influences on behavioral disinhibition. *American Journal of Medical Genetics, 96,* 684–695.

Zajonc, R. B. (1993). The confluence model: Differential or difference equation. *European Journal of Social Psychology, 23,* 211–215.

Zonderman, A. B. (1982). Differential heritability and consistency: A reanalysis of the National Merit Scholarship Qualifying Test (NMSQT) California Psychological Inventory (CPI) data. *Behavior Genetics, 12,* 193–208.

Zubenko, G. S., Hughes, H. B., & Stiffler, J. S. (2002). D2S2944 identifies a likely susceptibility locus for recurrent, early-onset, major depression in women. *Molecular Psychiatry, 7,* 460–467.

Author Index

Subject Index

9237

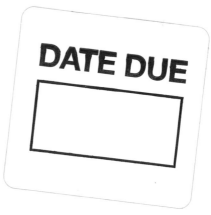

DATE DUE